OPERATIVE TECHNIQUES IN

LAPAROSCOPIC COLORECTAL SURGERY

Conor P. Delaney MD, MCh, PhD, FRCSI, FACS
Professor and Chief, Division of Colorectal Surgery
Vice-Chairman, Department of Surgery
Director, Institute for Surgery and Innovation
University Hospitals of Cleveland
Case Western Reserve University
Cleveland, Ohio

Paul C. Neary, MD, FRCSI (Gen)
Consultant Colorectal Surgeon
Department of Surgery
Adelaide and Meath Hospital,
Incorporating the National Children's Hospital
Dublin, Ireland

Alexander G. Heriot, MA, MD, FRCS (Gen), FRCSEd
Honorary Senior Lecturer
Department of Surgery
St. Vincent's Hospital, Melbourne University
Consultant Colorectal Surgeon
Department of Surgical Oncology
Peter MacCallum Cancer Centre
St. Andrews Place, East Melbourne, Victoria, Australia

Anthony J. Senagore, MD, MS, FACS, FASCRS
Professor and Chairman
Department of Surgery
University Medical Center at the Medical University of Ohio
Toledo, Ohio

Lippincott Williams & Wilkins
a Wolters Kluwer business
Philadelphia · Baltimore · New York · London
Buenos Aires · Hong Kong · Sydney · Tokyo

Acquisitions Editor: Brian Brown
Managing Editor: Julia Seto
Project Manager: Dave Murphy
Manufacturing Manager: Ben Rivera
Associate Director of Marketing: Adam Glazer
Design Coordinator: Risa Clow
Production Services: Laserwords Private Limited
Printer: Gopsons Paper Limited

© 2007 by LIPPINCOTT WILLIAMS & WILKINS, a Wolters Kluwer business
530 Walnut Street
Philadelphia, PA 19106 USA
LWW.com

Printed in the USA

Library of Congress Cataloging-in-Publication Data
Operative techniques in laparoscopic colorectal surgery / Conor Delaney . . . [et al.].
   p. ; cm.
  Includes bibliographical references and index.
  ISBN-13: 978-0-7817-6634-0
  ISBN-10: 0-7817-6634-6
  1. Colon (Anatomy)—Endoscopic surgery. 2. Rectum—Endoscopic surgery.
3. Laparoscopic surgery. I. Delaney, C. P. (Conor Patrick).
  [DNLM: 1. Colon—surgery. 2. Rectum—surgery. 3. Laparoscopy—methods. WI 650 O61 2007]
RD544.O64 2007
617.5′54707545—dc22

2006014744

10 9 8 7 6 5 4 3 2

Dedication

To my wife Clare for her constant support, and to my children Peter and Michelle for making life so much fun

C.P.D.

To my beautiful young daughters Rachael and Rebecca that give me sunshine everyday and most of all to my wife Geraldine who is my true strength and love

P.C.N.

In memory of my mother, Cynthia

A.G.H.

To my wife Patricia for her love and friendship, and our children Antonio and Christina for allowing me to learn from them

A.J.S.

Table of Contents

Preface

Although laparoscopic colorectal surgery has now been performed for 15 years, uptake into the surgical community has been slower than anticipated. One of the primary reasons for this delay has been the significant learning curve that laparoscopic colectomy requires.

Laparoscopic colorectal surgical training methods involve the use of a variety of laboratory-based courses, and technical lectures, and it is becoming recognized that teaching laparoscopic colectomy is a multistep process. Surgeons who wish to learn laparoscopic colectomy come with differing levels of experience. No matter what the level of experience, what all these surgeons require is familiarity with the operative steps of laparoscopic colectomy.

This book is a new venture to complement programs that teach laparoscopic colectomy. The book facilitates that process by helping students of laparoscopic colectomy develop the pattern-recognition skills required to perform this technique safely and successfully. Each chapter starts with a detailed textual description of procedures. Chapters are accompanied by a DVD that has been edited to display key steps of the laparoscopic portions of each surgical procedure. The book offers a reference databank of edited operative videos for each colonic surgery commonly performed laparoscopically.

The book starts with chapters describing the background information required to perform laparoscopic colorectal surgery. Operative videos are then divided into several groups. The first section presents videos of each component step used for colorectal procedures. Each is shown in detail with accompanying written text and a voice-over description of the procedure. The three basic surgeries of ileocecectomy, right colectomy, and sigmoid colectomy are shown in extensive detail with accompanying written text and a voice-over describing the procedure being performed. The final sections provide means of dealing with some intraoperative difficulties during laparoscopic colorectal surgery, and other useful techniques.

This should be a useful resource for residents and fellows in training, surgeons who are attending courses in laparoscopic colorectal surgery, and surgeons who are at an early stage of integrating this technique into their practice.

Conor P. Delaney
Paul C. Neary
Alexander G. Heriot
Anthony J. Senagore

Acknowledgment

The authors would like to thank the following for their excellent technical support.

Brian Hetsler and Fred Tribout, Department of Minimally Invasive Surgery, Cleveland Clinic Foundation
Gary Coffey, Department of Surgery,
University Hospitals of Cleveland, Cleveland, Ohio

Traditional Postoperative Management and Fast-track Care Pathways

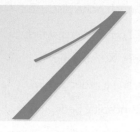

Traditional Postoperative Management and Fast-track Care Pathways

There have been remarkable developments and improvements in surgery but despite this, surgical intervention represents a significant assault upon the human body. Cuthbertson identified the impact of surgery on normal physiology and described the posttraumatic hyper catabolism, which has been termed the *stress* response. This homeostatic disequilibrium is manifested by the neuroendocrine system through a systemic metabolic response, which results in physiologic and psychological changes in the patient. The stress response to surgery causes an increase in the demands on various organs, and this increased demand contributes to the development of postoperative organ dysfunction. This may cause impairment in pulmonary and cardiovascular function, fluid retention, and gastrointestinal ileus, along with fatigue, muscle weakness, and pain.

The traditional postoperative management of patients undergoing major abdominal surgery utilizes the routine use of nasogastric tubes and abdominal drains, prolonged bladder catheterization, copious analgesia, and prolonged abstinence of oral intake until the patient has begun to pass flatus, as there is resolution of the intestinal ileus. This management results in patients having to stay in a hospital for anything between 5 to 10 days following major abdominal surgery such as colonic resection; the average stay in many centers is over 10 days. Such results are greatly impacted by the surgeon, and the culture from which these data come; in some countries, the length of stay has traditionally been close to 3 weeks after bowel resection.

The length of the hospital stay following major abdominal surgery has significant clinical and economic implications, both at the individual patient level and at the national level. For the individual, a longer stay increases the risk of nosocomial infections and complications. From a national perspective, Medicare data from 1999 to 2000 in the United States reported a mean postoperative stay of 11.3 days, following major intestinal or colorectal resection. This was derived from 161,000 resections in patients of >65 years of age, and corresponded to a total of 1.8 million bed days with an estimated overall postoperative care cost of $1.75 billion per annum.

The importance of the reduction of the length of stay has become increasingly recognized and is reflected by published literature. Between 1985 and 1990 there were

13 publications in the literature relating to the length of stay, although none discussed any methods to shorten this. From 1995 to 2000 there were 122 publications, which included multiple prospective randomized and cohort comparisons with the aim of reducing the length of stay. There are a variety of issues encouraging a reduction in the length of stay in hospital. The availability of resources, such as hospital beds, in first world healthcare systems is being reduced as the size of the elderly population increases. There is reduced financial reimbursement to hospitals and physicians, combined with increasing costs. Finally, there is an increasing emphasis on the standardization and optimization of the quality of care; this is easier to demonstrate on the background of defined management protocols and discharge criteria, which are an essential component of strategies to reduce hospital stay.

TUBES, DRAINS, AND CATHETERS

A variety of approaches have been developed to reduce hospital stay. Preoperative assessment and detailed preoperative information to be given to the patient is essential. This is combined with patient education, standardized preoperative orders, and information about postoperative expectations. A meta-analysis of the use of nasogastric tubes after intestinal surgery assessed 26 trials with a total of 3,694 patients. Fever, atelectasis, pneumonia, and the number of days to the toleration of diet were significantly less without a nasogastric tube. There was increased vomiting and abdominal distension when nasogastric tubes were not used, but no other complication was increased with a reinsertion rate of 5%. The early removal of the urinary catheter also allows improved mobilization during recovery from surgery. Drains are used selectively, such as for ultralow anterior resections, and are removed early at between 24 and 48 hours postoperatively.

PAIN CONTROL

The issue of pain control has been addressed in a number of ways. The management of the patient's pain is essential to encourage early mobilization. It has been considered that the prevention of pain, and hence the reduction of the neurophysiological and biochemical consequences of pain may be more beneficial than the treatment of established pain. This "preemptive analgesia", however, has failed to show any effect on postoperative pain in a systematic review of more than 80 randomized clinical trials; nor has the suggested physiologic benefit demonstrated an evidence-base improvement in clinical benefit.

Opioid analgesia is the most commonly used form of analgesia, although it does have well recognized side effects, including nausea and ileus. Intravenous patient-controlled analgesia may allow lower doses to be administered, and patients can begin oral analgesia as soon as their ileus has begun to resolve. Epidural-based anaesthesia has been shown to provide effective pain relief, and may be better than intravenous administration for the control of pain in the first 24 to 48 hours. It has been suggested that the use of local anesthetic rather than opioid-based infusions through the epidural may improve gastrointestinal function. Kehlet has suggested that epidural analgesia is a prerequisite for enhanced recovery programs following major surgery; however, Zutshi et al. reported a randomized controlled study comparing intravenous patient-controlled analgesia with epidural analgesia in the context of an enhanced recovery program, and showed no difference in the time of discharge or patient satisfaction.

Pain in the postoperative period represents the operation of several different nociceptive mechanisms and hence the utilization of several different treatment modalities has the potential to optimize analgesia and minimize side effects. The combination of nonsteroidal anti-inflammatory drugs (NSAIDs), with opioids and paracetamol, has been demonstrated to improve analgesia in several randomized studies. NSAIDs such as ketoralac can be given intravenously until there is a resolution of the ileus, and can reduce the total narcotic dose required. As soon as the patient is able to tolerate oral fluids, analgesic requirements can be managed with combined oral analgesia, utilizing oral NSAIDs such as diclofenac with oral analgesia such as oxycodone. Trials comparing laparoscopic versus open colorectal resections have also demonstrated a consistent reduction in postoperative analgesic requirements, as a consequence of the difference in incision size.

ILEUS

Postoperative ileus may be defined as a transient cessation of coordinated bowel motility after surgical intervention, which prevents the effective transit of intestinal contents and/or tolerance of oral intake. This definition was recently ratified at a Consensus Conference of a multidisciplinary panel titled the Postoperative Ileus Management Council, which was held in New York in 2005.

Factors causing postoperative ileus include inhibitory sympathetic reflexes initiated from the site of injury, local intestinal inflammatory responses, and opioids. It has been suggested that epidural anaesthesia may contribute to a reduction in ileus, but the relative role of epidural anaesthesia versus early oral nutrition and mobilization has not been resolved. Early enteral nutrition has been shown to reduce postoperative morbidity, and eliminating the routine use of nasogastric tubes in combination with instituting early oral nutrition has demonstrated a significant reduction in hospital stay following colorectal surgery. The application of laparoscopic surgery with reduced handling of the small bowel may also reduce the duration of ileus as compared to open surgery. In the author's practice, patients begin oral fluids immediately after surgery, and are offered a soft diet the morning after surgery.

Fluid management in the postoperative period can have a significant impact on recovery after surgery, including the duration of ileus. The administration of large volumes of fluid should be avoided as it has the potential to prolong ileus, as well as increase the risk of cardiac and pulmonary complications. Lobo et al. demonstrated in a randomized controlled trial that salt and water restriction after elective colonic surgery hastened return of the gastrointestinal function.

The pharmacologic manipulation of ileus is an area of ongoing research. A number of drugs have demonstrated promising results in the reduction of the duration of ileus and postoperative nausea, and this is likely to be an important area of ongoing research. Taguchi et al. reported a reduction in time to enteral diet and time to discharge with the use of ADL 8-2698, a peripheral mu-opioid receptor antagonist. A multicenter trial evaluating the use of alvimopan after abdominal surgery has shown a significant reduction in the time of gastrointestinal recovery, particularly after intestinal resection.

A combination of these efforts, including the provision of effective dynamic pain relief, the reduction of surgical stress responses and organ dysfunction, along with early mobilization and oral nutrition, has been synthesized into the concept of "fast-track" or "enhanced recovery" postoperative care. Fast-track surgical programs have been applied to a range of surgical procedures and there have been a number of studies assessing colonic resection, comparing fast-track to standard management following open colorectal resection. Basse et al. from Kehlet's unit in Denmark, a pioneer of fast-track surgery, compared 130 patients having conventional care following colonic surgery with an equivalent number receiving fast-track care, with a reduction in time to defecation, morbidity, and hospital stay, the latter being reduced from 8 to 2 days. Delaney et al. reported the application of a standardized fast-track protocol named the CREAD (Controlled Rehabilitation with Early Ambulation and Diet), for patients undergoing colonic resection without routine epidural use. In a randomized trial between CREAD and conventional postoperative management, there was a significant reduction in the median length of stay from 5 days to 3.8 days in the CREAD group, with no difference in pain score or patient satisfaction. The same group showed that a similar protocol was also applicable to complex reoperative pelvic surgery with a reduction in the length of stay and no increase in complications. There has been concern that the use of a fast-track protocol might result in increased readmissions after discharge. This has not been publicized by any study, and Kiran et al. reported that unplanned readmission was unpredictable and was not precipitated by a shorter length of stay at the primary admission.

The application of laparoscopic surgery to colorectal resection may be easily integrated into fast-track protocols and has the potential to further reduce the length of stay. A case-matched comparison of clinical and financial outcomes after laparoscopic or open colorectal surgery reported a significant reduction in the length of stay and in hospital costs in the laparoscopic group. This must be contrasted with a randomized study by Basse et al. who compared open fast track with laparoscopic fast-track colonic resection and reported no difference in the length of stay between the groups and a median length of stay of 2 days. Although this subject requires further study, most randomized trials comparing open and laparoscopic approaches to colorectal surgery have demonstrated a reduction of hospital stay in the order of 2 days.

In conclusion, fast-track protocols can be applied to patients undergoing either open or laparoscopic colorectal surgery with a significant reduction in hospital stay. There is no obvious increase in complications or readmission, and patient satisfaction is equivalent. Pharmacologic manipulation and the increased application of laparoscopic techniques are likely to be integrated into future fast-track protocols.

Chapter TWO

Development of Laparoscopic Colorectal Surgery

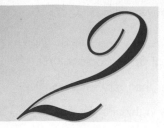

Development of Laparoscopic Colorectal Surgery

A | TECHNICAL ADVANCES MAKING PROCEDURES FEASIBLE

The advent of laparoscopic surgery has had a tremendous impact on gastrointestinal surgery over the last 20 years. The first laparoscopic cholecystectomy was performed in 1987, and within a few years there was widespread adoption of the laparoscopic technique as the standard care for the treatment of gallbladder disease. The first laparoscopic colonic resection was performed in 1991, but the uptake of the approach has been dramatically slower and it is only over the last few years that it has become more commonplace. One explanation for this has been the concern of using a laparoscopic approach for colorectal malignancy, which has only recently been resolved by the publication of the survival results of the Clinical Outcomes of Surgical Therapy (COST) trial, which reported equivalence between the open and laparoscopic approaches in terms of recurrence and survival. A recent editorial that accompanied the publication of the COST study in the New England Journal of Medicine was titled "Laparoscopic resection for colon cancer—the end of the beginning?".

An additional explanation is that laparoscopic colorectal resection is technically a more difficult procedure than laparoscopy for gallbladder disease, obesity, or gastroesophageal reflux, and that technical advances over the last decade have greatly facilitated the development and uptake of laparoscopic colorectal surgery.

Laparoscopic colorectal resection necessitates a number of steps, which differ from other laparoscopic procedures such as cholecystectomy or Nissen fundoplication. It requires significant dissection in multiple abdominal quadrants, division of large vessels, and bowel division and reanastomosis. Developments in video imaging with improvements in resolution and camera design have greatly facilitated the ability to identify the anatomy and allow dissection. Quality video imaging is essential for all laparoscopic surgery, necessitated by the obvious lack of tactile sensation other than through the laparoscopic instruments, but particularly for more advanced procedures such as laparoscopic colorectal surgery.

The division of large vessels is an almost unique requirement of laparoscopic colorectal surgery, and simple diathermy is inadequate for anything other than very small vessels. A standard laparoscopic clip applicator can be used, but difficulty in thinning the vessel attachment down can complicate clip application. Developments in stapling technology, such as an endoscopic vascular stapler with 2.5 mm staples, allows the division of large arteries with good hemostasis.

Endoscopic staplers with 3.5 mm or larger staples can be used to divide the bowel if intracorporeal division is required. This technology has been further improved by the ability to angulate reticulating staplers. This facilitates the division of the rectum within the pelvis in situations where a straight stapler would simply not reach, and has permitted developments such as low rectal division just at the anal canal.

There have also been significant developments in systems to allow energy delivery. This is important for tissue and vessel division and dissection. Precise hemostasis is important, as blood impairs the identification of tissue planes and causes image deterioration by greatly reducing the available light. Dissection can be performed with standard diathermy, but more extended dissections necessitating extensive intracorporeal mesenteric division such as subtotal colectomy may be greatly facilitated by energy delivery systems. Ultrasonic dissectors (Ultracision, Harmonic scalpel) and advanced diathermy technology (LigaSure) have been important technologic developments, which have been used to facilitate laparoscopic colorectal surgery. The LigaSure is a high-energy coagulator that can seal vessels of up to 7 mm. It seals the vessel by changing the collagen structure, and provides a reliable and safe hemostatic seal.

Considerable dissection is required to mobilize the colon and there is a significant learning curve. There have been developments such as handports, which may be inserted into a 7 to 9 cm incision while maintaining a pneumoperitoneum to allow a hand to be inserted into the abdominal cavity to aid dissection. This technology permits tactile sensation, restores depth perception, and has been proposed as a technique to shorten the learning curve for laparoscopic colorectal surgery and reduce the conversion rate. Published evidence has not conclusively shown clinical or training benefits over standard laparoscopic approaches, and this technology is still being evaluated.

B | BENIGN VERSUS MALIGNANT DISEASE

Concerns that the laparoscopic resection of colorectal malignancy may have inferior results to open resection in terms of recurrence and overall survival has been a significant factor in the delay in the uptake of laparoscopic colorectal surgery. Nevertheless, there has been increasing evidence over the last decade that the results of laparoscopic surgery for malignancy are at least equivalent to that of open surgery in terms of recurrence and survival.

Initial concerns over laparoscopic surgery for colorectal cancer were related to an unusual pattern of local wound recurrence, which was even noted in Dukes A patients, with the most number of recurrences in the first year. The possibility that a laparoscopic approach altered the pattern of recurrence, resulting in port site metastases, generated significant concern. It is likely that the problem was related to technical factors and poor oncologic principles in the early development of the laparoscopic techniques, as the incidence of port site metastases has declined to an incidence similar to that of wound recurrence rate in open surgery, generally <1%. Comparative trials of open and laparoscopic approaches have shown no difference in wound or port site recurrence rate. Ziprin et al. in a review of the incidence of port site metastases reported that despite concerns from early studies, there did not appear to be any increased risk of port site metastases with laparoscopic surgery. The publication of a number of multicenter randomized controlled studies has confirmed this.

Cancer-free survival is by necessity a long-term outcome, hence initial observations as to whether the laparoscopic approach was oncologically equivalent focused on potential surrogate markers such as specimen equivalence between the two approaches. Milsom et al. and Lacy et al. both reported no difference in resection margin involvement and lymph node yield in the resected specimen between open and laparoscopic approaches. Initial survival outcomes began to appear from a series of patients undergoing laparoscopic resection. Hartley et al. reported no difference in local or distant recurrence from 109 patients undergoing either open or laparoscopic resection in a prospective nonrandomized study. Fleshman et al. retrospectively reviewed 372 patients who had undergone laparoscopic resection, and reported that their 3-year survival was similar to that reported for open resection.

A number of multicenter randomized trials were set up in the United States, United Kingdom, and Europe, but prior to these being mature, a number of single-center randomized trials reported the survival results between open and laparoscopic resection. In 2002, Lacy et al. reported a randomized trial of over 200 patients undergoing open or laparoscopic resection of colon cancer. It demonstrated an improvement in cancer-related survival in the laparoscopic group, and subgroup analysis demonstrated that this was due to an improved outcome in patients with Stage III disease. Leung et al. reported a randomized trial from Hong Kong of rectosigmoid tumors, and demonstrated identical recurrence and survival between open and laparoscopic approaches.

The results from adequately powered multicenter randomized trials remain the gold standard for evidence, and it was inevitable that these were required before a more generalized acceptance of a laparoscopic approach for cancer. The Clinical Outcomes of Surgical Therapy (COST) Study Group published in 2004, reported the results of a randomized trial between laparoscopic and open surgery for colonic carcinoma. It randomized 872 patients and reported no difference in either recurrence (16% vs. 18%), wound recurrence (<1% in both groups), or in 3-year survival (86% vs. 85%) between the laparoscopic and open group, respectively. There was no difference in complications, but the laparoscopic group demonstrated shorter postoperative recovery and a reduction in analgesic requirements. Survival data from other large randomized trials, the COlon carcinoma Laparoscopic or Open Resection (COLOR) trial in Europe, and the Conventional versus Laparoscopic Assisted Surgery In Colorectal Cancer (CLASICC) trial in the United Kingdom are awaited, although early data shows no difference in recurrence. The results of the COST study led to a joint statement from The American Society of Colon and Rectal Surgeons and Society of American Gastrointestinal Endoscopic Surgeons (SAGES) *"Laparoscopic colectomy for curable cancer results in equivalent cancer-related survival to open colectomy when performed by experienced surgeons. . . . Based upon the COST trial, pre-requisite experience should include at least 20 laparoscopic colorectal resections with anastomosis for benign disease or metastatic colon cancer before using the technique to treat curable cancer."* An editorial accompanying the publication of the COST study deftly caught the current situation and was entitled "Laparoscopic resection for colon cancer—the end of the beginning?" The changes in practice for surgery of colorectal cancer over the next decade are likely to be significant.

Laparoscopy for benign colorectal disease has a different set of hurdles. Obviously the concerns over oncologic equivalence to open surgery are irrelevant, but unfortunately, due to the inflammatory nature of the disease process in the case of diverticular disease or inflammatory bowel disease, benign disease is technically more challenging.

The boundaries for a laparoscopic approach have progressively been pushed back over the last decade.

Rectal prolapse requires rectal mobilization, and with the exception of resection rectopexy, no bowel resection or anastomosis, and is hence an ideal procedure to perform laparoscopically. Solomon et al. reported the only randomized controlled trial comparing laparoscopic and open resection with an improvement in the length of stay, analgesic requirement, and cost in the laparoscopic group.

There have been multiple reports of laparoscopic resection for diverticular disease. Purkyastha et al. have reported a meta-analysis, comparing open and laparoscopic approaches for diverticular disease, and have shown a reduction in complications and in the length of stay in the laparoscopic group. Diverticular fistulas have been managed successfully laparoscopically, although the conversion rate is higher.

The spectrum of disease presentation for Crohn's disease can be wide, but ileocolic disease remains the most common indication for surgical intervention. Ileocolic resection has been shown to be suitable for a laparoscopic approach with a reduction in complications and in the length of stay. Complicated disease, including ileosigmoid fistulas, can also be managed laparoscopically but requires greater surgical experience, and has a higher conversion rate. Colonic resections may be performed for both Crohn's disease and ulcerative colitis as the indications for a laparoscopic approach, including ileoanal pouch surgery. As with malignant disease, laparoscopy looks likely to become the approach of choice for benign colorectal disease in an increasingly large proportion of cases in the future.

C | TRAINING AND INITIAL CASE SELECTION

TRAINING

Laparoscopic colorectal surgery is the most significant technical development in colorectal surgery over the last decade, and is likely to have a significant impact on the training and delivery of colorectal surgery.

Laparoscopic surgery has developed as an integral component of general surgery since the early 1990s with the introduction of laparoscopic cholecystectomy, and has necessitated a change in the approach to surgical training. There are fundamental differences in the skills required for laparoscopic surgery as compared to open surgery. The use of long instruments with the associated fulcrum effect and the lack of tactile sensation combined with a two-dimensional image of which only the tips of the instruments are visible, provide a different set of challenges to the operating surgeon and to training individuals in laparoscopic techniques. The wide acceptance of more routinely performed laparoscopic abdominal procedures such as cholecystectomy or appendicectomy has made the development of laparoscopic skills amongst trainee surgeons more usual, but laparoscopic colorectal surgery provides a number of specific difficulties which makes it more challenging to learn and perform.

Laparoscopic colorectal surgery involves operating in between one and four abdominal quadrants. It is necessary to divide vessels of a significant size and often remove a large specimen. The formation of a bowel anastomosis is often required, and there are a variety of different operations that can be performed, a significant proportion of these involving malignant pathology. The introduction of laparoscopic cholecystectomy was associated with an increase in surgical morbidity in terms of bile duct injury, and the increased complexity of laparoscopic colorectal surgery raises the possibility of a similar scenario, unless surgeons undergo adequate training. Training surgeons in laparoscopic colorectal surgery does pose difficulties in terms of case numbers, as it has been recognized that there is a measurable learning curve in acquiring the required skills to reach a steady state in terms of technique, time, and complications. Tekkis et al. assessed the learning curve for right- and left-sided laparoscopic colonic resections. Using cumulative sum (CUSUM) analysis and adjusting for case mix, they reported that 55 cases were required for right-sided resections and 62 for left-sided resection. This was consistent with other studies which reported a learning curve of between 30 and 70 cases. One problem is that the average general surgery resident graduates with an average of 1 abdominoperineal resection, 7 rectal resections, and 20 to 30 colon resections logged during their training. Once in practice, the average general surgeon performs approximately ten colorectal resections per year, which makes the completion of a laparoscopic learning curve difficult. Currently, training in advanced colorectal surgery has been attained by undertaking a colorectal fellowship after the completion of residency training. The availability of laparoscopic colorectal training, however, has been restricted to a limited number of specialized centers. This is changing, particularly following the publication of the Clinical Outcomes of Surgical Therapy (COST) study in 2004, as more colorectal surgeons are proactively seeking training, but this is likely to contribute to some delays in a more generalized uptake. Laparoscopic colorectal workshops that utilize both animal and human cadaver models have been developed, often in conjunction with industry support, to facilitate training and try to shorten the learning curve. However, training with experienced surgeons who consistently perform a significant number of laparoscopic colorectal procedures remains the optimum way to acquire the required skills.

CASE SELECTION

Appropriate case selection is an essential component of surgical practice and this remains true for laparoscopic colorectal surgery. An inappropriate selection of patients is likely to result in an increased rate of complications and conversion to open procedures. A number of factors have been identified that influence the likelihood of conversion to an open procedure. Body mass index (BMI), American Society of Anesthesiologists (ASA) score, surgeon experience, the type of resection (left more difficult than right), and the presence of intra-abdominal abscess or enteric fistula have all been shown to be important factors that influence the likelihood of conversion. The requirement to convert is not necessarily detrimental, as Casillas et al. have shown that the outcome is equivalent provided the decision to convert is made early. This is in contrast to the COST study, which reported a worse outcome in patients who required conversion to open surgery. The impact of specific factors is relative, as a number of series have reported good results following laparoscopic colorectal procedures in patients with high BMI and in patients with enteroenteric fistulas, although this involved experienced laparoscopic colorectal surgeons in both cases.

Therefore, ideal cases to start on to help climb the learning curve are those that allow the surgeon the opportunity to go through the simple steps of right and left hemicolectomy. Patients with a low BMI should be chosen, who have not had prior abdominal surgery. A cecal polyp is a good option, although cancer precautions must be taken, as up to 20% of cases can harbor invasive malignancy. Similarly, terminal ileal Crohn's disease may be suitable. If complications or other difficulties arise in either case, then the patient should be converted to open surgery, knowing that a conversion is far safer than progressing through a complex case when inadequately experienced. For left colectomies, polyp and simple uncomplicated recurrent diverticulitis are likely to be the best options.

Chapter THREE

Instrumentation and Setup

Instrumentation and Setup

A | OPERATING ROOM REQUIREMENTS

Many procedures have developed into routine laparoscopic procedures; however, the basic operating room equipment and setup should be familiar to most general surgeons. The key issues that must be considered are positioning of monitors for viewing by the entire surgical team, easy access to carbon dioxide for insufflation, and proximity to the generators for cautery or other energy instruments. An electric operating bed with stirrups for the legs is optimal so that the patient can be easily airplaned during the procedure for the different positions required for access.

Monitors are probably best placed on booms to allow full motion for positioning at locations that provide good visualization by the operating team. It is possible to use carts for the same purpose; however, they typically occupy more floor space and limit mobility in the room.

Carbon dioxide may be supplied from a central location and piped into the room. This approach is superior because it diminishes issues related to temperature differences of the gas, which may increase fogging. Most surgeons use individual tanks that carry the risk of running out of gas. If this approach is used, a spare tank should always be present in the room to avoid unnecessary delays or unexpected loss of visualization.

There are a variety of new energy modalities that may be used in laparoscopic surgery. These include monopolar and bipolar cautery, harmonic scalpels, and devices like the LigaSure. Each of these devices requires a generator that must be located close enough to allow the cords to reach the field. Once again, placing these devices on a single boom is the most efficient means of providing access to the field and to the circulating nurse. However, carts can be used in a similar manner at the expense of the operating room floor space.

A final point to consider is the ability to take advantage of the digital video technology to allow for electronic recording of the procedure. Digital video disc (DVD) technology is readily available and a recorder can be placed on a cart or a boom with the light source or the video output for the camera, to allow the surgeon to record the entire procedure on video. Alternatively, high-resolution printers can be used to print still pictures of portions of the surgical procedure.

B   SURGICAL INSTRUMENTS

The development of laparoscopic surgery dates back over 100 years, and the instrumentation available continues to improve with time. The rudimentary development of endoscopy dates far earlier than this. In 1585, Aranzi used focused sunlight to examine the nasal cavity and in 1706, the term *trocar* was coined to describe a three-faced instrument enclosed in a metal cannula. In 1901, Georg Kelling performed experimental laparoscopy on a canine model in Berlin and by 1929, Kalk was pioneering the use of laparoscopy with an angled viewing lens. Ruddock performed diagnostic laparoscopy in the United States in 1934, and several years later Janos Veres introduced the "Veres needle." This was a dedicated laparoscopic instrument used for creating a pneumothorax for subsequent minimally invasive surgery.[1] Modifications of the Veres needle are still used today by many surgeons to create the pneumoperitoneum before the trocar insertion. In 1971, Hasson introduced a blunt-tipped operating trocar that permitted surgeons to use a direct vision "open" technique to create the pneumoperitoneum.[2] Modified versions of the Hasson port are established as being the principal method used by most surgeons today and is indeed the technique used in the authors' own colorectal laparoscopic practice for creating the operating pneumoperitoneum.

Imaging systems have also evolved in tandem with the pioneering efforts of the early laparoscopic surgeons. The introduction of the videoscope and expansion of imaging quality from initial single chip to three chips to digitalized image capture at the camera head has progressively offered the surgeon an enhanced view of the surgical field.

The improvements in image quality have been essential in permitting further expansion of the number of surgeries previously considered only the remit of an "open" approach now established as routine in laparoscopic surgery. In 1983, Semm in Germany reported a laparoscopic appendicectomy; in 1987, Mouret performed a laparoscopic cholecystectomy with a "videoscope"; and in 1991, Jacobs reported 20 cases of laparoscopically performed colectomies.

The technology behind the dissecting instrumentation has also rapidly developed since these early surgical cases. Initially, electrocautery was the predominant dissecting modality; however, in the early 1990s, ultrasonic dissectors and lasers were introduced. Currently, operating surgeons have a wide variety of instrumentation available, as both the speed and size of the surgical instruments have evolved. In this chapter, we review the basic requirements of instrumentation for effectively undertaking laparoscopic colorectal surgery. The nature of the instruments required and the complete "operating instrument set" are discussed on an individual basis for the main colorectal surgeries.

BASIC LAPARO-SCOPIC INSTRUMENTS

It should be noted that nearly all the instruments that are described are currently available, both in reusable format and as a disposable model. The rationale for using a disposable version of a reusable instrument may be related to surgeon preference, hospital and operative economics, and, particularly, case load volume for each surgical practice.

Laparoscopic ports

Laparoscopic operating ports provide the surgeon access to the laparoscopic operating environment (see Figure 3B.1). The instrument consists of an outer sleeve termed a *cannula* and an introducer termed a *trocar*. The trocar may be sharp or blunt tipped. Once the instrument is introduced through the abdominal wall, the trocar is removed and the port is secured either by suture or by nature of the threads that are built onto

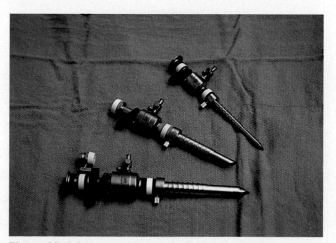

Figure 3B.1 Selection of Hasson ports, sizes and lengths.

the cannula. The basic requirements of the port are that it is easy to insert, ergonomically comfortable to use, permits ease of exchange of surgical instruments, does not dislodge from the abdominal wall once inserted, and does not cause surrounding tissue damage either from insertion, lateral conductance, or capacitance. There is a wide range of laparoscopic ports available in the market today. The port size required reflects the largest instrument that will be introduced through that operating port. In colorectal surgery, the largest instrument required is usually the endoscopic GIA used for bowel transection, but also considering the different diameters of staple cartridges of some manufacturers for larger staple height loads. Therefore, this requires a port size of 12 to 15 mm diameter. Available port sizes vary from this down through 10–12 mm, 5 mm, and 2 mm. As the imaging systems improve and surgical instruments also improve, the ongoing reduction in optimum port size required will also continue. The operating ports are now also available in varying lengths and this is sometimes useful to facilitate placement of an operating port through a large panniculus in obese patients.

Modified Hasson ports

The Hasson port consists of a blunt-tipped trocar that is used for creation of the pneumoperitoneum. It is used as a subumbilical access port for establishment of the pneumoperitoneum in our cases. The port is of 10 to 12 mm diameter and facilitates introduction of a 10-mm laparoscope. The cannula is designed with an associated external thread or screw to grip the fascia and prevent dislocation of the port during the procedure. There are a variety of modified Hasson ports in the market with variable designs of external thread mechanisms to ensure fixity of the port. In most models, the external thread is movable and this permits adjustment of the intra-abdominal cannula length, if required. Alternatively, a reusable port may be used as the trocar for the modified Hasson technique, simply requiring removal of the trocar from the port before insertion through the open wound.

Operating ports

The basic design of the operating ports mirrors that of the modified Hasson port. The size of the port varies and may be as small as 2 mm in diameter. The standard operating ports that we currently use for surgery are of 12-, 10-, and 5-mm diameter respectively. The introducing trocar is sharp to permit entry through the abdominal wall and many of the disposable instruments have a spring-loaded retractable tip guard that helps in reducing the possibility of inadvertent visceral injury. The internal chambers of all laparoscopic ports are designed to enable instrument removal and reintroduction without losing the established pneumoperitoneum. This is achieved either by a sequential trumpet valve or a flapper valve mechanism. Some of the current ports may also be used to accommo-date a selection of instrument sizes from 12 to 5 mm. These ports have a superficial seal that expands to accommodate the instrument. In other systems, an additional "lid" may be placed over the port to "downsize" the port orifice. The wide selection of laparo-scopic ports that is available reflects the evolving technology and competition in this aspect of the market.

Bowel graspers and long instruments

Bowel graspers are designed to permit the surgeon to hold and manipulate the bowel without damaging the serosa or, at worst, incurring an inadvertent enterotomy (see Figure 3B.2). The bowel grasper must therefore not have a sharp edge and preferably exert the line of pressure on the bowel wall in a uniform manner, distributed over the length of the instrument. The graspers have an operating handle piece connected to a shaft and end with the grasping forceps themselves. The instruments vary in length from a standard 36-cm shaft to the longer instruments that measure 43 cm in length. The operating handle comprises one fixed arm and a second movable arm, with a grip mech-anism similar to a scissors. The handle piece connects to a centre rod that traverses the shaft of the instrument and attaches to the operating tip. The rod in the shaft moves as the handle is opened or closed and the graspers at the end of the shaft open and close correspondingly. The instruments should be nonconductive and the coating should not have a high reflective nature. This is to avoid conduction injury and impairment of the laparoscopic videocamera light detecting system. The grasping jaws permit dual opening and the shaft may have a "toggle" to permit a 360-degree rotation in its longitudinal axis. The graspers may be traumatic or atraumatic in nature and fenestrated or solid in design. It is essential that the surgeon has a long bowel grasper (43-cm shaft) and a long-shafted laparoscopic scissors packed separately as these may be useful in obese patients, deep

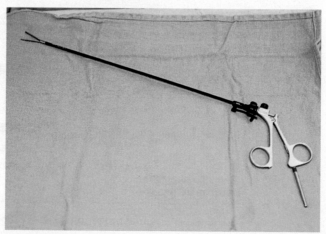

Figure 3B.2 Bowel graspers.

in the pelvis and in mobilization of the splenic flexure. Some instruments equivalent to those used in open colorectal surgery have also been introduced into the laparoscopic field, such as the laparoscopic Babcock clamp. Although some surgeons prefer these instruments, they are not a prerequisite component in our standard colorectal laparoscopic operating set.

Scissors

There is a variety of reusable and disposable laparoscopic scissors currently available in the market (see Figure 3B.3). A standard laparoscopic scissors comprises a 5-mm diameter shaft and curved blades of 16 mm length. The blades should be sharp and permit both tissue transection and blunt dissection if used when closed. The jaws open 8 mm in span and may be rotated through 360 degrees by use of a toggle located near the grasping handle. The tips of the scissors should be blunt and this avoids inadvertent transgression across dissecting planes when making blunt dissection. The blunt tip also potentially reduces any possible enteric injury when the instrument is being introduced and removed through the 5-mm operating ports. The cutting jaws may be curved as in a Mayo scissors or straight. A curved scissors is preferable for pelvic dissection. The degree of curvature of the scissor tips is a point of personal preference; however, it should be of significant degree to permit easy angulation in the pelvis and near the splenic flexure. The functional grip of the scissors is designed similar to the grasping forceps with a dual lever handgrip and variable length shaft (31–43 cm). The scissors also have an attachment for electrocautery and the shaft is insulated to prevent coagulation injury to adjacent structures.

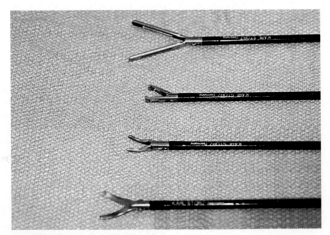

Figure 3B.3 Examples of laparoscopic scissors.

Traumatic graspers

The use of traumatic graspers in laparoscopic bowel surgery is not recommended because of the concern of tearing the intestine or mesentery; however, there are certain traumatic instruments that are specifically required for elements of this complex surgery. The laparoscopic Allis forceps comprises a 5-mm diameter shaft, a hinged operating handle, and traumatic grasping jaws. The instrument permits rigid holding of the anvil of a circular stapler to reapproximate the stapling mechanism when one is performing a left-sided colorectal anastomosis. The instrument may also be used to aid in retracting the soft tissue that gathers around the circular stapling gun as it is introduced through the rectal stump. It functions well in approximating the anastomosis; however, it may tear the bowel wall if not used judiciously.

A Maryland grasping forceps should be included in the laparoscopic colorectal operating instrument set. This again should be with an insulated operating handle. The instrument fits down a 5-mm operating port and is commonly used in other laparoscopic procedures such as cholecystectomy. The Maryland grasping forceps is a traumatic grasper due to its serrated edges. It should not be used to perform significant bowel mobilization, as the standard bowel graspers are more forgiving. The Maryland forceps is useful in providing pinpoint grasping of a divided/bleeding vessel. The vessel may then be coagulated, if the size and location permit this. The Maryland forceps, consequently, also has an electrocautery attachment available for monopolar electrocautery. The tips of the Maryland forceps may be curved or even angulated. This permits efficacy in grasping tissues or vessels that are hard to access with the straight bowel graspers.

Retractors

The development of laparoscopic retractors has led to a variety of designs and techniques applicable to the spectrum of advanced laparoscopic procedures. Many of the devices are disposable and need a 10-mm operating port to introduce them. The variety of disposable designs includes a fan retractor that may be articulated, a paddle retractor, or a "snake" retractor. All the retractors have been used previously in upper gastrointestinal surgery and are often more applicable to retraction of a fixed organ such as the liver rather than small bowel viscera. In colorectal surgery, most small bowel mobilization is performed independent of instrument retraction but rather by gravitational displacement. Occasionally in certain patients, in whom obesity, adhesions, or anesthetic requirements limit steep Trendelenburg position, the use of a bowel retractor is necessary. The optimum retractor for colorectal surgery should fit down a 5-mm operating port, be capable of capturing and holding the small bowel away from the operative field, and not interfere with the surgical instruments. The cost of the instrument and the ergonomics of its use should also be favorable to the surgeon. Each of the traditional retractors does not fulfill these requirements completely. The fan retractor works by rotating the hand piece control to open the individual blades of the fan. This is a linear configuration and the final appearance is similar to fingers of a hand. The blades of the fan retractor may cause inadvertent organ injury and should be closely observed when the blades are being opened and eventually closed. The paddle retractor is operated in a similar manner; however, the functional retractor end piece is a continuous barrier mesh. The small bowel tends to slip around the margins of the instrument resulting in migration into the operating field. The "snake" retractor fits down a 5-mm operating port and is closed by dialing the functional hand piece similar to the fan retractor. The retractor closes in a triangular configuration without any central barrier mesh. The result is that the small bowel may be herniated through the center of the instrument and require repositioning on a regular basis. As the instrument is opened to form the triangular retractor, the tip of the instrument approximates the origin of the triangle. This may catch small bowel loops and cause iatrogenic injury if not used carefully.

ENERGY-BASED DISSECTING INSTRUMENTA-TION

Ultrasonic-based dissectors

The principle underlying ultrasonic-based laparoscopic instruments involves the conversion of high frequency ultrasonic waves to a mechanically based energy delivery system. The components of the operating system are an ultrasonic wave generator, a piezoelectric transducer, and an operating blade. The generator is an AC power supply that uses a microprocessor to control the vibration of the transducer at 55.5 kHz. Longitudinal sound waves are generated at a constant frequency of 55,500 cycles per second. The hand piece then conducts this energy through a collection of piezoelectric ceramics located between metal cylinders. This results in a magnetostrictive transducer that creates mechanical vibrations in the functional operating blade. The generated mechanical vibration is conducted directly to the operating tip. The generator is a reusable machine and the shaft diameter is 5 mm. The functional tip appears similar to a scissors with the vibrating or functional blade being the mobile aspect of the scissors. Dissection through tissues necessitates elevation of the tissue under tension as the ultrasonic instrument divides the target tissues. The size of the vessels that may be safely divided with these energy systems is up to 5-mm in diameter. From a surgical viewpoint the instrument may be used through a 5-mm operating port. Activation of the ultrasonic energy is controlled by using a "foot-pedal" or a "contact button" on the hand piece itself. There is a degree of rotational mobility of the shaft itself that approaches 360 degrees.

Electrocautery-based instrumentation

The mechanism of action of electrocautery-based instrumentation differs entirely from that of the ultrasonic-based instruments. The LigaSure vessel sealing system uses a combination of pressure and thermal energy to seal the selected vessels. The operating system consists of a generator and operating hand piece. The instrument is available with 10- and 5-mm diameter shafts. The hand piece comprises a functional handgrip with a locking mechanism, once the handles are closed. This may be released if the surgeon wishes to regrasp the selected tissue. The instrument is controlled using a "foot-pedal" and once the pedal is depressed the generator will provide an acoustic signal to indicate the commencement of coagulation. Once the instrument senses that the vessel is ligated, the pitch of the acoustic signal indicates completion of the vessel sealing. A trigger on the hand piece is then used to release a cutting blade that transects between the sealed tissues. The result is a sealed and divided vessel. The instrument may be used through a 5-mm operating port and the vessel size that can be divided is up to 7-mm in diameter. For larger vessels, many surgeons apply a double 'firing' of the LigaSure having an area of cautery proximal to the area that is divided as an additional assurance of hemostasis. The instrument may be rotated using the hand piece toggle and provides functional rotational movement of the blades. The 5-mm shaft is connected to the operating tips and these grasp, ligate, and subsequently divide the tissue chosen. The hand piece is disposable in nature and attaches to the mobile generator. The surrounding thermal injury to tissue is limited to approximately 2 mm on an average for most LigaSure instruments.

INDIVIDUAL CASE REQUIRE-MENTS

Combined with the standard laparoscopic surgical instruments it is necessary to have a selection of open retractors and forceps in the "set." The following table outlines a standard colorectal operating instrument set for a segmental colectomy. The surgeon should have the "extra-long" instruments packed separately (one 43-cm shaft scissors and one 43-cm shaft bowel grasper) as these will not be used in all cases. In cases of ileocecectomy where there is a bulky mesentery, further artery or Kocher forceps may be required for extracorporeal division of the ileocolic mesentery.

SEGMENTAL LAPARO-SCOPIC COLECTOMY

Open instruments

Sponge holding forceps (for sterilizing the skin before incision)	2
Ball-and-socket towel clips	2
Bachus towel clips	2

Standard toothed dissecting forceps	1
Adson toothed dissecting forceps	1
DeBakey nontoothed dissecting forceps	1
Standard nontoothed dissecting forceps	1
Spencer Wells curved artery forceps	5
Heiss 9″ artery forceps	5
Metz scissors 7″	1
Curved Mayo scissors 6.5″	1
Crilewood needle holder 6″	1
Mayo needle holder 8″	1
Kocher forceps	5
Babcock clamp	4
Allis forceps	2
Lagenbeck retractors	2

Laparoscopic instruments

Zero degree laparoscope and electrical and optical cables	1
Bowel graspers (36 cm)	3
Maryland forceps (36 cm)	1
Scissors (36 cm)	1
Wound protector (variable size)	1
Suture passer for wound closure	1

Used in left side colectomy primarily

Allis forceps (36 cm)	1

Available but not routinely used

Bowel grasper (43 cm)	1
Scissors (43 cm)	1

REFERENCES

1. Veres J. Nues instrumentzur ausfuhrung von brust—oder bauchpunktionen und pneumothoraxbehandlung. *Dtsch Med Wochenschr.* 1938;40: 1480–1481.
2. Hasson HM. A modified instrument and method for laparoscopy. *Obstet Gynecol.* 1971;110: 886–887.

C FINANCIAL IMPLICATIONS OF LAPAROSCOPIC COLECTOMY

Although laparoscopic colectomy is slowly gaining acceptance, it is difficult to demonstrate cost effectiveness of the procedures based on the available literature. Cost effectiveness of laparoscopic colectomy can occur only under the following conditions: (i) The surgeon and surgical team have fully ascended the learning curve; (ii) careful assessment and implementation of required technology in the operating room; (iii) full implementation of standard fast-track care programs for optimal postoperative recovery (information presented in Chapter 1). Coupling an old-fashioned postoperative care plan with nasogastric tubes, delay in resuming diets, and high dose narcotic analgesia will diffuse any potential benefits of a minimally invasive colectomy. The resource consumption must be balanced between the higher costs consumed in the operating room and the significant potential for less resource use during the hospital stay. The COlon Carcinoma Laparoscopic or Open Resection (COLOR) trial has demonstrated that when these contingencies are not met there can be a significant disadvantage for laparoscopic colectomy.

OPERATING ROOM COST

The major source of excessive cost in the operating room for laparoscopic colectomy is prolonged operative time. This is primarily a function of the steep learning curve. The specific standard steps to the various procedures have been presented throughout this book and will not be repeated. However, it can be clearly demonstrated that all experienced groups have developed clear-cut steps that benchmark progress, decrease procedural variability, and shorten the time for the procedure or do not delay timely conversion. The ascension of the learning curve results in operative times that approximate open colectomy duration or at worst do not exceed those times by >60 minutes. Procedures with durations of >5 hours will have a difficult time indeed of ever becoming cost effective.

Conversion by itself will not directly lead to increased costs, provided a reasonable rate of conversion (<15%) is maintained by the team. In addition, conversion should occur as the result of accurate assessment of failure to progress, rather than intraoperative complications leading to urgent conversion. Our team has consistently demonstrated that converted patients do not consume excessive additional resources when managed with standard optimal recovery programs. In fact, converted patients will not progress any differently than patients in whom open colectomy is started in the beginning. The use of a standard medial-to-lateral approach offers early completion of anatomical identification and vascular ligation that are typically the most significant contributors to failure or progress. Recent work by our group has demonstrated that 50% of conversions occur due to failure of these two steps that typically require <15 minutes and occur before opening most of the disposable laparoscopic equipment.

Consumption of technology in the operating room is another variable source of cost, and an issue that can quickly take on a life of its own if not frequently assessed by the team. It is clear that certain tools are required to gain access to the abdominal cavity, provide hemostasis, securely ligate and divide the vascular supply, and divide supporting tissue or bowel. A variety of trocars are available that range from completely reusable, to resposable (partially reusable), to one-time use equipment. The determination of which set to use requires local economic knowledge because the trade-off costs are acquisition, cleaning, breakage, and repackaging for reusable components versus acquisition, warehousing, and timely availability in the operating room. In general, higher volume hospitals are more likely to maintain skilled staff and turnaround times that make reusable trocars the better option.

A variety of devices can be used to safely and efficiently provide hemostasis during dissection. In general, we feel that monopolar cautery is the most effective in terms of speed and coagulation for most clinical scenarios. If the surgeon maintains dissection within natural anatomic planes, large blood vessels are rarely encountered which would require attention. This can be supplemented by reusable bipolar cautery forceps for unusual clinical situations. Vascular ligation will require something capable of securely replacing suture material. For major pedicles, options include clips (slower, multiple applications, nondividing), harmonic scalpel (limited to smaller vessels, not major pedicles), LigaSure (ligates and divides major pedicles), or endoscopic staplers (ligates and divides major pedicles). The cost decision for these devices is dependent on the number of large vessels encountered and alternative usage of the instrument. As discussed in the preceding text, most dissections should occur in a bloodless plane so the relative advantage of other energy-delivering devices becomes problematic compared to the cautery. For left-sided resections that require division of only the internal mesenteric artery (IMA) pedicle, a single application of a vascular stapling cartridge is far less expensive (by 70%) than advanced energy equipment because the stapler will be required later in the procedure for the bowel transection. If a multisegmental colectomy is performed, which requires transection of multiple major pedicles, it is more advantageous to consider the use of the LigaSure or other energy source, because it can be used for the dissection and transection steps of the procedure while reducing instrument exchanges. In addition, the device is less expensive than 3 to 4 stapling cartridges.

Reusable dissecting equipment and other hand pieces are readily available and offer unique solutions for most clinical scenarios. It does not seem likely that reusable instrumentation can be anything but the obvious choice for most laparoscopic colectomy cases. Our team has standardized a set to include: Three atraumatic bowel graspers, two Allis clamps, two scissors, and a retracting device. Many of these kits have been used for more than 200 cases without need for repair or replacement (aside from scissor sharpening).

As for the current debate regarding hand-assist versus two-handed laparoscopic techniques, the verdict is still out. The putative benefits of shorter operative times and lower conversion rates have yet to be verified by experienced groups. In addition, the acquisition price for the various devices ranges from US $450 to $700 and must therefore be balanced against some other direct cost. If the only benefit is modest reductions in operative times, it will be difficult to yield cost efficiency because a minimum reduction of 1.5 hours would be required to allow an additional case to be performed in that same operating room. In addition, there is a disadvantage to the surgeon as a hand-assist case should be billed using the open current procedural terminology (CPT) code rather than the laparoscopic code.

HOSPITALIZATION COST SAVINGS

The potential sources for cost savings during the recovery phase are contingent on utilizing a fast-track care plan that will provide an optimal recovery program for the patient. This will allow the patient to take advantage of smaller wounds, less pain, and decreased physiologic stress to shorten the hospital stay. In addition, because these patients typically transition off parenteral medications earlier and move to a normal diet there is less cost for intravenous medications. Furthermore, these patients have far fewer instances of ileus, postoperative fevers, urinary tract infections, and wound infections. The result is a far lower utilization rate of laboratory studies, diagnostic radiology, microbiology evaluation, and nasogastric drainage. Implications are obvious to the institution in terms of resource consumption in these areas. However, as discussed in the preceding text, all of these benefits can be erased by injudicious use of operating room equipment or failure to use an enhanced recovery program.

**PAYER COST
SAVINGS**

Under Part A of the US Medicare fee schedule, colectomy patients are assigned to either Disease Related Group (DRG) 148 (colorectal resection with complications) or DRG 149 (colorectal resection without complications) with significant reimbursement implications ($149 to $8,310; $148 to $20,291). Our group compared 100 consecutive patients from a prospective database, undergoing laparoscopic segmental colectomy and assigned to DRG 148, to a case-matched group of patients undergoing open colectomy. Significantly, more patients in the laparoscopic group of patients were assigned DRG 148 solely due to preoperative comorbidities (LAP-62 vs. OPEN-21; $p < 0.0001$). Equally importantly, more patients in the OPEN group were classified as DRG 148 solely due to postoperative complications (LAP-22 vs. OPEN-42; $p < 0.0001$). Mean direct hospital costs were significantly less for laparoscopic patients (LAP-$3,971; OPEN-$5,997; $p = 0.0095$) and resulted in a 33% reduction in direct cost to the institution. Therefore, under a prospective payment system, laparoscopic colectomy can significantly effect DRG assignment and cost of care for the payer and provider. It simultaneously frees up additional capacity for the institution, which presents an opportunity to further increase revenue while improving patient access to services.

Chapter FOUR

Key Operative Steps

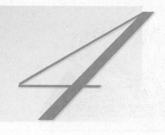

Key Operative Steps

A	POSITIONING AND BASIC PORT INSERTION ⟲ DVD

PATIENT POSITIONING

The patient is placed supine on the operating table on a beanbag with pneumatic compression devices. The operating room (OR) table needs to be one that can have the leg section removed, or partially removed and moved out of the way. General anesthesia is induced, and then an orogastric tube and Foley catheter are inserted.

The arms are tucked at the patient's side. For morbid patients in whom an arm must be kept out because of OR table size, or for cases in which the anesthesiologist needs access, an arm may be kept out on the side of the colon being removed (left arm out for sigmoid colectomy). This is because the assistant will need space to stand beside the surgeon for most of the procedure.

The legs are placed in Dan Allen or Yellowfin stirrups. The legs are kept in position with the knees slightly flexed, and the hips straight or even slightly extended (see Figure 4A.1). The patient's perineum needs to be at the lower end of the bed so that a stapler may be inserted for anastomosis. The beanbag is now aspirated, fixing the patient in position. In our practice, shoulder straps are generally avoided for fear of brachial plexus injury. Chest strapping with adhesive tape is rarely done.

The abdomen is then prepared with antiseptic solution and draped routinely. We tend to use disposable drapes with pockets, which allow the cords to be positioned out of the way of the surgeons.

INSTRUMENT POSITIONING

Cables for CO_2, light, cautery, and other energy sources are somewhat dependent on the setup of the individual ORs. Generally, it is best to have them come off at the cephalad end, so the surgeon and assistant are not trapped beside the patient.

Monitor positions are described in each relevant chapter, for each type of colectomy. Generally, the primary monitor is placed at the side of the patient up toward the

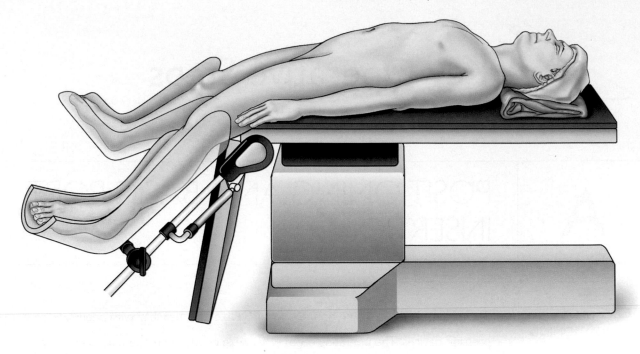

Figure 4A.1 The patient is positioned on the table in Dan Allen stirrups.

patient's feet, at approximately the level of the hip. The secondary monitor is placed on the opposite side of the patient at the shoulder level, and is primarily for the assistant during the early phase of surgery and port insertion (see Figure 4A.2).

The operating nurses' instrument table is placed between the patient's legs, and is mobile to permit the surgeon to come between the patient's legs for total colectomies, or for mobilization of splenic flexure. There should be sufficient space to allow the surgeon to move from either side of the patient to between the patient's legs, if necessary.

UMBILICAL PORT INSERTION

Umbilical port insertion is performed using a modified Hasson approach. A vertical 1 cm subumbilical incision is made. This is deepened down to the linea alba, which is then grasped on each side of the midline using Kocher clamps. A scalpel (No. 15 blade) is used to open the fascia between the Kocher clamps and a Kelly forceps is used to open the peritoneum, bluntly. It is important to keep this opening small (<1 cm) to minimize air leaks.

Having made entry into the peritoneal cavity, a purse-string suture of 0 polyglycolic acid is placed around the subumbilical fascial defect (umbilical port site) and a Rommel tourniquet is applied. A 10-mm reusable port is inserted through this port site allowing the abdomen to be insufflated with CO_2 to a pressure of 12 mm Hg. The camera is inserted into the abdomen and an initial laparoscopy is performed, carefully evaluating the liver, small bowel, and peritoneal surfaces. The remaining ports are inserted as necessary (see Figures 4A.3–4A.6).

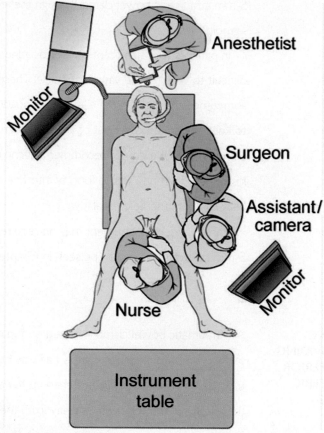

Figure 4A.2 Operating room setup for right side procedures.

B | LOW INFERIOR MESENTERIC ARTERY LIGATION 💿

SETUP

The assistant and surgeon are on the patient's right side, with the assistant at shoulder level. The patient is rotated with the left side up and right side down, to approximately 15 to 20 degrees tilt, and often as far as the table can go. This helps to move the small bowel over to the right side of the abdomen. The patient is then placed in the Trendelenburg position. This again helps gravitational migration of the small bowel away from the operative field. The surgeon then inserts two atraumatic bowel clamps through the two left-sided abdominal ports. The greater omentum is reflected over the transverse colon so that it comes to lie on the stomach. If there is no space in the upper part of the abdomen, one must confirm that the orogastric tube is adequately decompressing the stomach. The small bowel is moved to the patient's right upper quadrant, allowing visualization of the inferior mesenteric pedicle. This may necessitate the use of the assistant's

5-mm atraumatic bowel clamp through the left lower quadrant to adequately tent up the sigmoid mesentery.

In patients with significant obesity or adhesions in the upper quadrants, it can be difficult to visualize the vascular pedicle. These adhesions may need to be lysed, or, sometimes, the insertion of a left upper quadrant port allows use of another retractor to keep the small bowel out of the way. Such instruments are often left in place for some time, so we do not recommend clamping the intestine, but rather using a closed instrument to gently push a loop of intestine out of the way, and, if necessary, coming back to check the field regularly.

Rarely, a fourth instrument may be required, and, if so, we tend to use a malleable 5-mm retractor, which can be seen in Chapter 7F.

DEFINING AND DIVIDING THE INFERIOR MESENTERIC PEDICLE

An atraumatic bowel clamp is placed on the rectosigmoid mesentery at the level of the sacral promontory, approximately half way between the bowel wall and the promontory itself. This area is then stretched up toward the left lower quadrant port, stretching the inferior mesenteric vessels away from the retroperitoneum (see Figure 4B.1). In most cases this demonstrates a groove between the right, or medial side of the inferior mesenteric pedicle and the retroperitoneum. Cautery is used to open the peritoneum along this line, opening the plane cranially up to the origin of the inferior mesenteric artery, and caudally past the sacral promontory (see Figure 4B.2). A blunt dissection is then used to lift the vessels away from the retroperitoneum and presacral autonomic nerves (see Figure 4B.3). The ureter is then located under the inferior mesenteric artery (see Figure 4B.4). If the dissection is in the correct plane, the ureter should be just deep to the parietal peritoneum, and just medial to the gonadal vessels. Care must be taken not to dissect too deep and injure the iliac vessels. If the psoas tendon is encountered, the plane of dissection is too lateral.

If the ureter cannot be found, it is probably elevated on the back of the inferior mesenteric pedicle, and one needs to stay very close to the vessel, not only to find the ureter but also to protect the autonomic nerves. If the ureter still cannot be found, dissection from a cranial direction needs to be done, which is usually made into clean tissue allowing the ureter to be found. If this fails, a lateral approach can be performed (see subsequent text). This usually gives a fresh perspective to the tissues, and the ureter can often be found quite easily. In very rare cases the ureter still may not be found. We do not use routine ureteric stents, so the options at this stage include conversion to open surgery, or insertion of ureteric stents. We do not proceed if the ureter cannot be defined.

Having defined the inferior mesenteric pedicle, it is thinned out by dissecting the adipose tissue away (see Figure 4B.5). For benign disease, a low ligation may be performed, preserving the left colic artery and perhaps improving collateral blood supply. Cautery is then used to open a window in the peritoneum, lateral to the inferior mesenteric vessels.

The vessel is then divided using a low ligation, and a clamp is placed on the origin of the vessel to control it if clips or other energy sources do not adequately control the vessel (see Figure 4B.6). In general, for a left colectomy a cartridge of the ENDO GIA stapler is used to divide the vessel. This helps minimise expenditure, as the stapler will anyway be required for division of the rectum. Laparoscopic clips or other energy sources may also be used.

Having divided the vessel, the plane between the descending colon mesentery and the retroperitoneum is developed laterally, out toward the lateral attachment of the colon, and superiorly, dissecting the bowel off the anterior surface of the Gerota's fascia up toward the splenic flexure.

C | HIGH INFERIOR MESENTERIC ARTERY LIGATION

SETUP

The assistant and surgeon are on the patient's right side, with the assistant at the shoulder level. The patient is rotated with the left side up and right side down, to approximately 15 to 20 degrees tilt, and often as far as the table can go. This helps to move the small bowel over to the right side of the abdomen. The patient is then placed in the Trendelenburg position. This again helps gravitational migration of the small bowel away from the operative field. The surgeon then inserts two atraumatic bowel clamps through the two left-sided abdominal ports. The greater omentum is reflected over the transverse colon so that it comes to lie on the stomach. If there is no space in the upper part of the abdomen, one must confirm that the orogastric tube is adequately decompressing the stomach to expel the gas. The small bowel is moved to the patient's right upper quadrant, allowing visualization of the inferior mesenteric pedicle. This may necessitate the use of the assistant's 5-mm atraumatic bowel clamp through the left lower quadrant to adequately tent up the sigmoid mesentery.

In patients with significant obesity or adhesions in the upper quadrants, it can be difficult to visualize the vascular pedicle. These adhesions may need to be lysed, or, sometimes, the insertion of a left upper quadrant port allows use of another retractor to keep the small bowel out of the way. Such instruments are often left in place for some time, so we do not recommend clamping the intestine, but rather using a closed instrument to gently push a loop of intestine out of the way, and, if necessary, come back and check the field regularly.

Rarely, a fourth instrument may be required, and, if so, we tend to use a malleable 5-mm retractor, which can be seen in Chapter 7F.

DEFINING AND DIVIDING THE INFERIOR MESENTERIC PEDICLE

An atraumatic bowel clamp is placed on the rectosigmoid mesentery at the level of the sacral promontory, approximately half way between the bowel wall and the promontory itself. This area is then stretched up toward the left lower quadrant port, stretching the inferior mesenteric vessels away from the retroperitoneum. In most cases, this demonstrates a groove between the right, or medial side of the inferior mesenteric pedicle and the retroperitoneum. Cautery is used to open the peritoneum along this line, opening the plane cranially up to the origin of the inferior mesenteric artery, and caudally past the sacral promontory. A blunt dissection is then used to lift the vessels away from the retroperitoneum and presacral autonomic nerves. The ureter is then looked for under the inferior mesenteric artery. If the ureter cannot be seen, and the dissection is in the correct plane, the ureter should be just deep to the parietal peritoneum, and just medial to the gonadal vessels. Care must be taken not to dissect too deep and injure the iliac vessels. If the psoas tendon is encountered, the plane of dissection is too lateral.

If the ureter cannot be found, it has usually been elevated on the back of the inferior mesenteric pedicle, and one needs to stay very close to the vessel, not only to find the ureter but also to protect the autonomic nerves. If the ureter still cannot be found, a cranial dissection needs to be done, which is usually made into clean tissue allowing the ureter to be found. If this fails, a lateral approach can be performed (see subsequent text). This usually gives a fresh perspective to the tissues, and the ureter can often be found quite easily. In very rare cases the ureter may still not be found. We do not use routine ureteric stents, so the options at this stage include conversion to open surgery, or insertion of ureteric stents. We do not proceed if the ureter cannot be defined.

The dissection is continued up to the origin of the inferior mesenteric artery that is carefully defined and divided using a high ligation, above the left colic artery (see Figures 4C.1 and 4C.2). This usually requires some dissection to clean the vessel of surrounding adipose tissue. A clamp may be placed on the origin of the vessel to control it, if clips or other energy sources do not adequately control the vessel. In general, for a left colectomy a cartridge of the ENDO GIA stapler is used to divide the vessel. This helps minimise expenditure, as the stapler will anyway be required for division of the rectum. Laparoscopic clips or other energy sources may also be used. The inferior mesenteric vein can also be divided, and this can be frequently achieved with the same stapler cartridge as is being used for the artery.

Having divided the vessels at the origin of the artery, the plane between the descending colon mesentery and the retroperitoneum is developed laterally, out toward the lateral attachment of the colon, and superiorly, dissecting the bowel off the anterior surface of the Gerota's fascia up toward the splenic flexure. This makes the inferior vein quite obvious and this vessel can also be divided just inferior to the pancreas (see Figures 4C.3–4C.5). This allows increased reach for a coloanal anastomosis with or without neorectal reservoir.

D | LIGATION OF THE ILEOCOLIC ARTERY 💿

SETUP

The patient is rotated with the right side up and left side down, to approximately 15 to 20 degrees tilt, and often as far as the table can go. This helps to move the small bowel over to the left side of the abdomen. The patient may be placed in the Trendelenburg position, although this is not always necessary for this step. The surgeon then inserts two atraumatic bowel clamps through the two left-sided abdominal ports. The greater omentum is reflected over the transverse colon so that it comes to lie on the stomach. If there is no space in the upper part of the abdomen, one must confirm that the oro-gastric tube is adequately decompressing the stomach. The small bowel is moved to the patient's left side, some remaining in the pelvis and upper abdomen, allowing visualization of the ileocolic pedicle. This may necessitate the use of the assistant's 5-mm atraumatic bowel clamp through the right lower quadrant to tent the ileal mesentery, medially and cephalad.

DEFINING AND DIVIDING THE ILEOCOLIC PEDICLE

A noncrushing bowel clamp is placed on the mesentery just at the ileocecal junction. This area is then stretched up toward the right lower quadrant port, stretching the vessel and also lifting it up from the retroperitoneum. In almost all cases, this demonstrates a sulcus between the medial side of the ileocolic pedicle and the retroperitoneum (see Figure 4D.1). Cautery is used to open the peritoneum along this line. A blunt dissection is then used to lift the vessel away from the retroperitoneum, opening the plane cranially up to the origin of the ileocolic artery from the superior mesenteric artery (see Figure 4D.2). Generally, the surgeon's closed left-hand instrument is passed behind the ileocolic pedicle and used to elevate the structures off the retroperitoneum. The right-hand instrument is used to dissect the retroperitoneum off the back of the ascending colon mesentery (see Figure 4D.3). Care is taken to make sure that the plane of dissection is anterior to the congenital layer of peritoneum lying over the retroperitoneum, duodenum, and ureter. As long as this layer is preserved and the dissection is anterior to the duodenum, we do not, as a routine, display the right ureter.

Cautery is then used to open a window in the peritoneum lateral to the vessel, and to thin out the tissues around the vessel. The vessel is then divided (see Figure 4D.4). A clamp is placed on the origin of the vessel to control it, if clips or other energy sources do not adequately control the vessel. When possible, clips are used to divide the vessel in an effort to minimize costs, as no other staplers will be necessary and as the right branch of the middle colic artery may be taken using the same stapler cartridge. Laparoscopic staplers or other energy sources may also be used. Having divided the vessel, the plane between the ascending colon mesentery and the retroperitoneum is developed laterally, out toward the lateral attachment of the colon, and superiorly, dissecting the bowel off the anterior surface of the duodenum and pancreas.

E | DIVISION OF THE UPPER RECTUM AND MESORECTUM

SETUP

At this stage of the surgery the inferior mesenteric vessels have been mobilized and divided, and the rectum has already been adequately mobilized to the point of transection. The surgeon and the assistant are on the patient's right side, with the assistant standing cephalad to the surgeon.

The assistant now grasps the rectosigmoid junction through the left lower quadrant port, and draws it up and out of the pelvis somewhat anteriorly (see Figure 4E.1). This gives the surgeon a nice view of the posterior and right lateral surfaces of the mesorectum and of the presacral space, and a final decision can be made whether the dissection is adequate on the right side.

Once the dissection is complete, the assistant draws the rectosigmoid out of the pelvis, without anterior displacement, and slightly to the left, giving the surgeon a good view of the right side of the mesorectum, and allowing the decision to be made about the distal site of transection. If the surgery is being performed for malignancy, a flexible endoscope may be inserted to confirm that there is an adequate distal margin.

Cautery is used to open the peritoneum, perpendicular to the site to be transected. An atraumatic bowel grasper is then used to open a plane between the rectum and the mesorectum, by advancing the instrument between the two structures and separating the jaws in an anteroposterior direction (see Figure 4E.2). This reduces bleeding by minimizing avulsion of small vessels off the back of the mesorectum. Stretching the rectum up out of the pelvis, and drawing it somewhat to the patient's left allows the instrument to be passed through perpendicularly at the correct level. Great care is taken so that the posterior surface of the rectum is not injured.

An ENDO GIA stapler is then inserted through the right lower quadrant port and is used to divide the rectum (see Figure 4E.3). Two firings are usually required. If one cartridge is adequate, it is usually because the patient has a small body habitus, or because the site of division is on the narrower sigmoid colon.

The bowel grasper is then passed completely behind the rectum. The left lateral peritoneum can be divided, and the second stapler cartridge is inserted and fired to divide the bowel.

The assistant now grasps the divided proximal end of the rectum and draws it anteriorly and to the left. This tents up the mesorectum and displays it so that the surgeon can divide it. Care must be taken so as not to injure the presacral fascia, left ureter, or left pelvic sidewall. Our practice is, usually, to use monopolar or bipolar cautery, although clips or other energy sources can be used (see Figure 4E.4). Before dividing the final strand of the mesorectum, the distal end is carefully examined for hemostasis, as once the mesorectum is completely divided the rectum retracts deep down into the pelvis (see Figure 4E.5).

F | LAPAROSCOPIC ANASTOMOTIC TECHNIQUES

COLORECTAL, COLOANAL, AND ILEOANAL ANASTOMOSES

For all of these procedures, the pathology has been exteriorized and resected, and a stapled anastomosis is to be performed. Our practice is to perform all anastomoses for diverticular disease, to the rectum. For this reason the distal bowel cannot be exteriorized through any abdominal incision, as leaving this much distal bowel would necessitate a colo-colic anastomosis.

After exteriorization and resection, the anvil of an EEA stapling device is inserted using a handsewn purse-string suture, and the bowel returned to the abdomen and the fascia closed. The abdomen is re-insufflated and the proximal colon is found.

Orientation is confirmed by following the cut edge of the mesentery, back to the retroperitoneum. Adequacy of reach is then determined by placing the colon with the anvil, into the pelvis (see Figure 4F.1). If it lies spontaneously, then anastomotic tension will usually be absent. If the colon keeps falling back into the upper abdomen, then further mobilization of the splenic flexure is required (see Chapter 4G).

The circular stapler is then inserted into the rectum and carefully advanced up to the apex of the rectal stump (see Figures 4F.2 and 4F.3). This may be surprisingly difficult, and needs plenty of lubrication. The stapler is closed and the anastomosis is done routinely (see Figures 4F.4–4F.7). It usually comes to lie about one third of the way down into the pelvis. The "doughnuts" are examined for completeness. The colon is gently grasped at about the level of the sacral promontory and the pelvis is filled with irrigating fluid (see Figures 4F.8 and 4F.9). The anastomosis is tested by distending the rectum with air, using a proctoscope or a bulb syringe. Anastomotic tension is assessed by placing an instrument behind the mesentery, just above the sacral promontory, and elevating the colon away from the retroperitoneum (see Figure 4F.10).

Occasionally, it may be difficult to get the stapler to reach the apex of the rectal stump. The use of plenty of lubricant is important. Advancing the instrument with a rotating movement also helps it to slide by some mucosal folds. Great care must be taken if any laparoscopic instrument is used to hold the rectal stump, as it can very easily perforate the stump or leave a tear in the serosa.

In some cases, it is not possible to get the stapler in position. Two options are available. One is to extrude the spike of the stapler on the anterior wall of the rectum and perform an end-to-side anastomosis. The second is to resect more rectum, going down to where the circular stapler has reached and using an extra cartridge of the ENDO GIA instrument. This permits a standard end-to-end anastomosis to be completed.

ILEOCOLIC AND SMALL BOWEL ANASTOMOSES

For right colectomy and small bowel resections, the bowel is mobilized and the vessels are ligated, but the resection is performed extracorporeally to expedite the procedure and reduce unnecessary use of consumables.

The right colon is thereby exteriorized, usually through a short midline wound having removed the subumbilical port. A wound protector is used in cases with neoplasia. The distal small bowel is assessed and the small bowel mesentery divided extracorporeally using 0 polygylcolate ties for hemostasis. In cases with a bulky ileal mesentery in Crohn's disease, suture ligation of the mesentery may be used. The bowel is divided with a GIA stapler and an Allis clamp is placed on the proximal end of the small bowel so that it is not lost back into the abdomen, and so that orientation of the mesentery is maintained.

Attention is now turned to the area for division of the colon. The colonic mesentery is divided with cautery. Pulsatile mesenteric bleeding is confirmed and the vessel is ligated with 0 polygylcolate suture ties. Again, the colon is divided with the GIA stapler. The specimen is now removed from the field and examined to confirm the pathologic findings, and the adequacy of proximal and distal margins. Our practice is to perform a side-to-side anastomosis with a GIA stapler, buttressing the crotch of the anastomosis with an interrupted 3/0 polygylcolate suture. The lumen of the anastomosis is inspected to make sure there is no internal staple line bleeding. The resulting opening from the GIA stapler insertion site is then closed with a transverse stapler. The exterior surface of the anastomosis is checked for hemostasis and then returned to the abdomen. The mesenteric window is not closed.

G | MOBILIZATION OF THE SPLENIC FLEXURE

SETUP

Splenic flexure mobilization is performed during sigmoid or left colectomy or anterior resection, or as part of a total colectomy. The medial approach to the splenic flexure is described in Chapter 5I. In practice, the approach may be a combination of medial and lateral approaches. In this chapter, we concentrate on the lateral approach that is commonly performed during sigmoid colectomy.

SPLENIC FLEXURE MOBILIZATION

Complete lateral mobilization of the left colon up to the splenic flexure is performed as an initial step, and is performed as a routine during sigmoid colectomy (see Figure 4G.1).

Next, the descending colon is pulled medially using an atraumatic bowel clamp in the right lower quadrant port and the scissors are moved to the left iliac fossa port. A 5-mm left upper quadrant port may be necessary, particularly in those with a very high splenic flexure, or in very tall or obese individuals. The lateral attachments of the left colon are divided and the colon dissected off the Gerota's fascia over the left kidney. Sometimes, long laparoscopic instruments may be required.

Once the lateral attachments of the colon have been freed as far as possible—sometimes this approach even allows the surgeon to come around and mobilize some of the transverse colon—it becomes necessary to move medially and enter the lesser sac. Some surgeons prefer to perform this as an initial step before lateral mobilization. To enter the lesser sac, the patient is tilted to a slight reverse Trendelenburg position. An atraumatic bowel clamp is inserted through the right upper quadrant port, and one through the left upper quadrant port if available. The assistant holds up the greater omentum toward its left side, like a cape. The surgeon grasps the transverse colon toward the left side using a grasper in the right lower quadrant port to aid identification of the avascular plane between the greater omentum and the transverse mesocolon (see Figure 4G.2). Diathermy scissors are used through the left lower quadrant port to dissect this plane and enter the lesser sac (see Figure 4G.3). The surgeon often moves to stand between the patient's legs for this part of the procedure. This dissection is continued toward the splenic flexure.

Following separation of the omentum off the left side of the transverse colon, connection to the lateral dissection allows the splenic flexure to be fully mobilized (see Figure 4G.4). The colon at the flexure is retracted caudally and medially, and any residual restraining attachments are divided.

H | MOBILIZATION OF HEPATIC FLEXURE

SETUP

The ascending colon would usually have been mobilized at this stage, using the retroperitoneal approach described in Chapters 4D and 5A. The surgeon and assistant are on the patient's left side, with the assistant cephalad to the surgeon.

MOBILIZATION OF THE HEPATIC FLEXURE

The assistant grasps the transverse colon with the atraumatic bowel clamp and draws it inferiorly. The surgeon grasps the distal ascending colon with the atraumatic bowel clamp in his right hand and exerts traction on the ascending colon, medially and inferiorly. This maneuver puts the hepatic flexure under tension and permits division of the gastrocolic ligament, using scissors and cautery (see Figure 4H.1). The surgeon continues to progress along this mobilization plane to draw the hepatic flexure inferiorly and medially (see Figure 4H.2). Care must be taken to avoid injury to the gallbladder and the second part of the duodenum during hepatic flexure mobilization due to their proximity to the dissection. The line of traction as the gastrocolic ligament is divided changes to more elevation of the ascending colon by the assistant and medial traction on the proximal transverse colon by the surgeon.

As this dissection continues, the area of prior retroperitoneal dissection after division of the ileocolic pedicle becomes apparent. Once this area has been entered, it becomes clear that the only remaining attachment is the lateral peritoneal attachment along the ascending colon (see Figure 4H.3). This area, the white line of Toldt, is divided using cautery. This line is divided right down to the base of the cecum, and it may even be able to completely mobilize the appendix and the base of the cecum to the midline from this direction. The colon is then dissected completely free from the underlying duodenum and retroperitoneum and reflected entirely to the midline (see Figures 4H.4 and 4H.5). This completes the hepatic flexure mobilization, using the lateral-to-medial approach.

Mobilization of the hepatic flexure can be difficult. In patients who are very obese, it can be hard to complete the ascending colon mobilization to the level of the hepatic flexure. In these cases, the release of the hepatic flexure can sometimes be facilitated by turning the patient to an anti-Trendelenburg position. Mobilization can sometimes be facilitated by inserting an instrument in the right upper quadrant. This additional port may provide additional traction on the hepatic flexure. The surgeon may find it more comfortable to stand between the patient's legs and use the two inferiorly placed ports as the main dissection instruments.

PORT SITE CLOSURE

Port sites are closed only when >5 mm in size. A reusable device, such as ENDO CLOSE, is the instrument of choice. The instrument is used to pass a 0 polyglycolic acid suture tie through the fascia, planning to have a 1-cm bite of tissue. The instrument is repassed on to the other side of the wound and the end of the suture is extracted (Figures 41.1 – 41.3). An extracorporeal knot is tied, closing the fascia.

The purse-string suture that is placed at the umbilical port site is tied to close the fascia at this site.

The subcutaneous spaces are then irrigated and the wounds are closed with subcuticular 4/0 polyglycolate sutures.

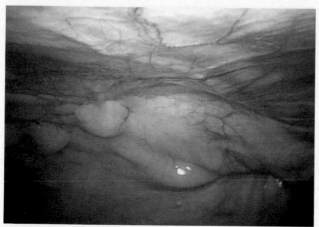

Figure 4A.3 The inferior epigastric vessels are carefully avoided.

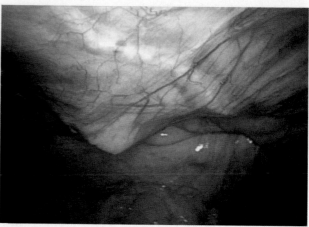

Figure 4A.4 The port is inserted with minimal force, rotating the blade to cut through the tissues.

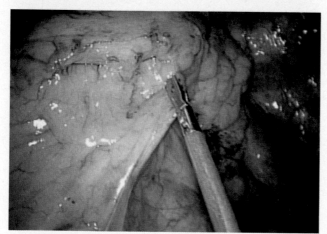

Figure 4A.5 The blade is guided lateral to the vessels.

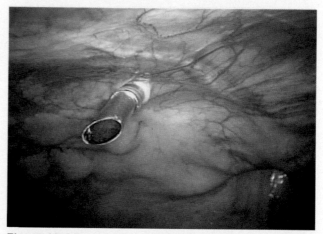

Figure 4A.6 The port lies lateral to the vessels.

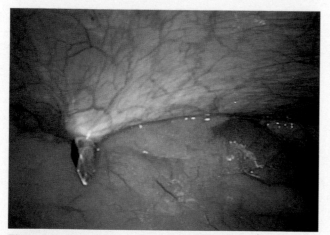

Figure 4B.1 Elevation of the sigmoid mesentery.

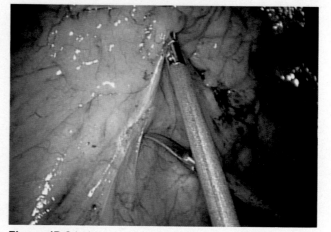

Figure 4B.2 Incising the peritoneum to define the inferior mesenteric vessels.

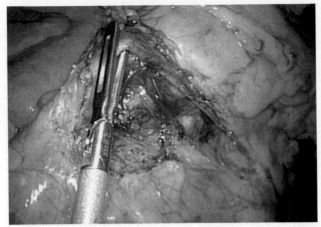

Figure 4B.3 Continuing to define the inferior mesenteric artery for low ligation.

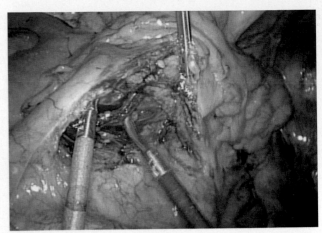

Figure 4B.4 Identifying the ureter prior to low ligation.

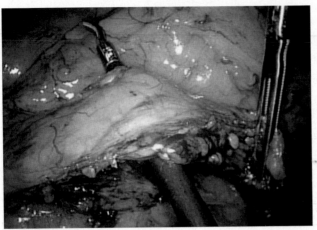

Figure 4B.5 Preparing the inferior mesenteric artery for division.

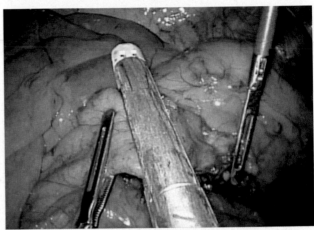

Figure 4B.6 Low ligation of the inferior mesenteric artery.

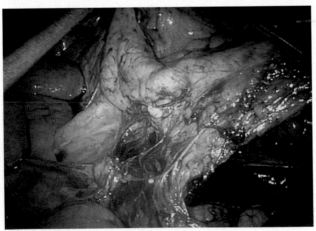

Figure 4C.1 The origin of the inferior mesenteric vessels is defined close to the aorta.

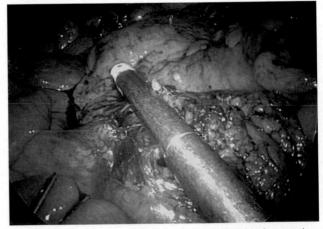

Figure 4C.2 The inferior mesenteric artery is divided approximately 1 cm distal to its origin.

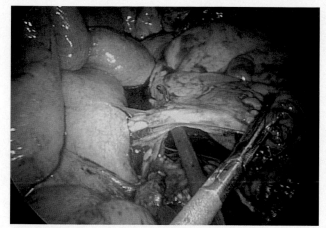

Figure 4C.3 The inferior mesenteric vein is defined close to the pancreas.

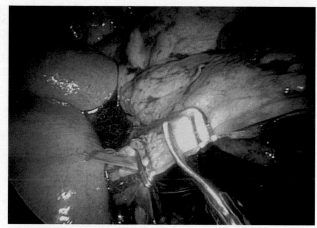

Figure 4C.4 The inferior mesenteric vein is divided.

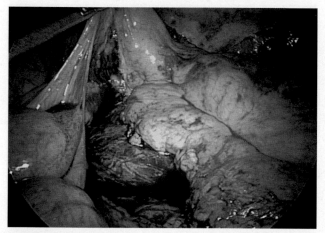

Figure 4C.5 The mesentery of the descending colon is completely mobilized.

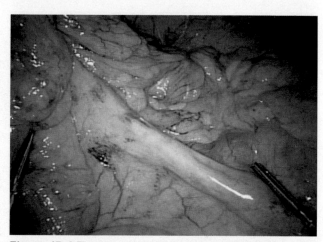

Figure 4D.1 The ileocolic pedicle and the duodenum.

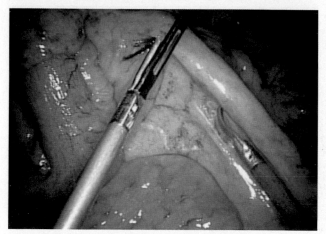

Figure 4D.2 Dissecting the ileocolic pedicle.

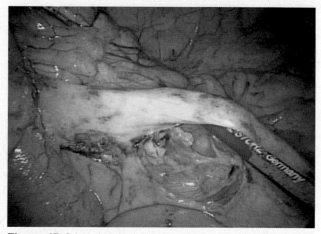

Figure 4D.3 Isolating the ileocolic pedicle.

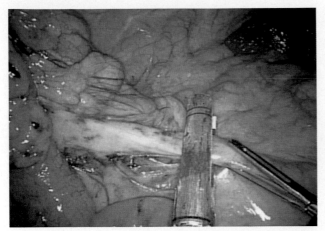

Figure 4D.4 Dividing the ileocolic pedicle.

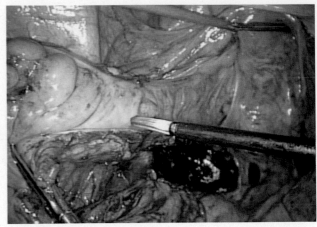

Figure 4E.1 The rectosigmoid junction is defined for rectal transection.

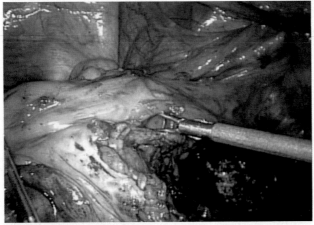

Figure 4E.2 A plane is developed between the rectum and the mesorectum.

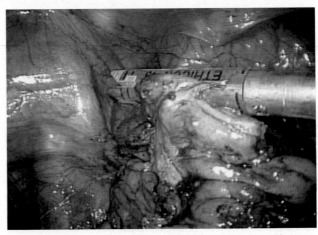

Figure 4E.3 The upper rectum is divided with endoscopic staplers.

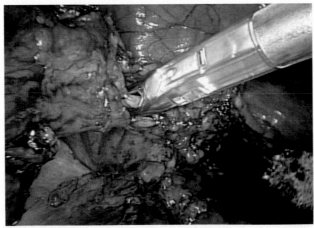

Figure 4E.4 The mesorectum is then divided using clips and cautery.

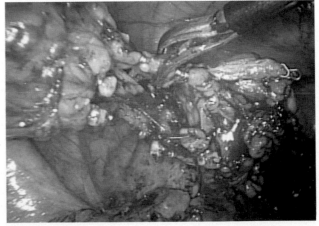

Figure 4E.5 The final part of the mesorectum is divided.

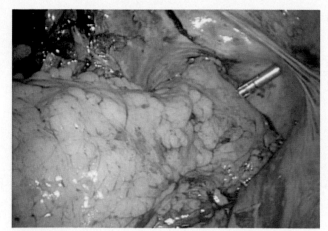

Figure 4F.1 Adequate reach of the proximal bowel is confirmed.

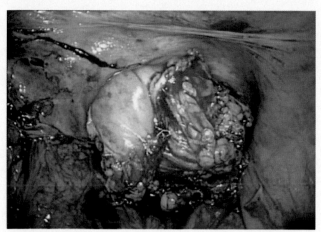

Figure 4F.2 The rectal staple line is visualized.

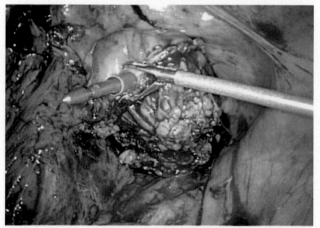

Figure 4F.3 The stapler is inserted into the rectum and the spike extruded through the staple line.

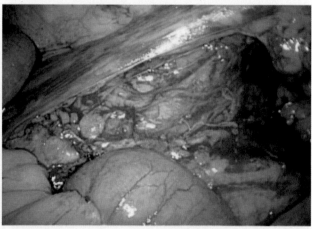

Figure 4F.4 The orientation of the proximal bowel is checked.

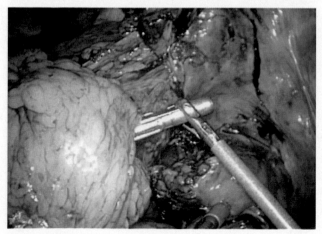

Figure 4F.5 The anvil is connected to the stapler.

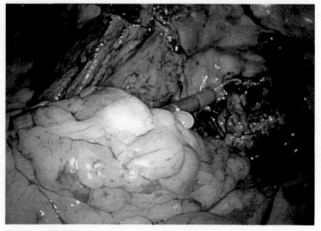

Figure 4F.6 The anastomosis is closed without torsion or tension.

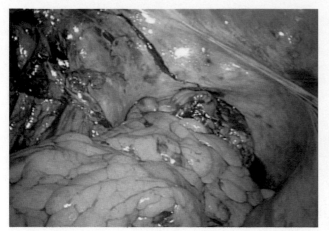

Figure 4F.7 The anastomosis is completed.

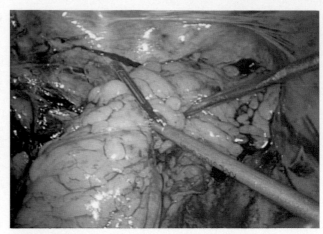

Figure 4F.8 The proximal bowel is closed off with a noncrushing clamp.

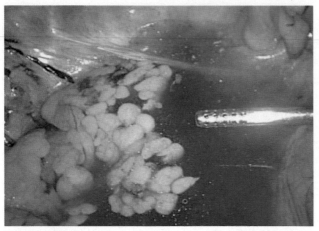

Figure 4F.9 The pelvis is filled with saline and the bowel is distended with air.

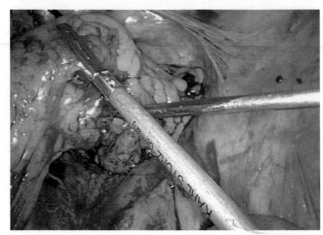

Figure 4F.10 The mesentery is elevated to make sure there is no tension on the anastomosis.

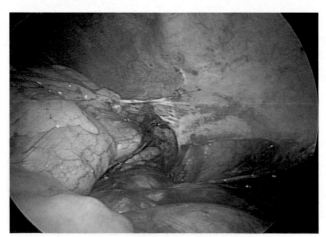

Figure 4G.1 Lateral mobilization of the descending colon is performed up to the splenic flexure.

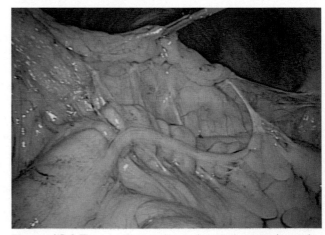

Figure 4G.2 The transverse colon and omentum are elevated.

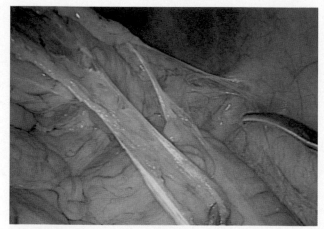

Figure 4G.3 The omentum is dissected off the transverse colon and the lesser sac is entered.

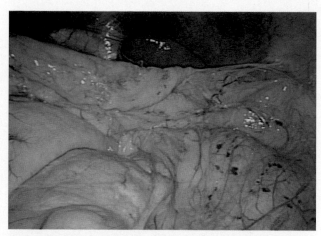

Figure 4G.4 The splenic flexure is completely mobilized, exposing the stomach, pancreas, and retroperitoneum.

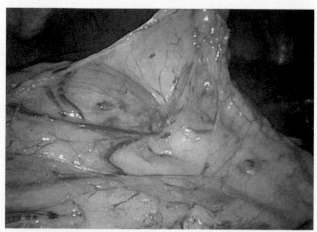

Figure 4H.1 The gastrocolic ligament is elevated to mobilize the hepatic flexure.

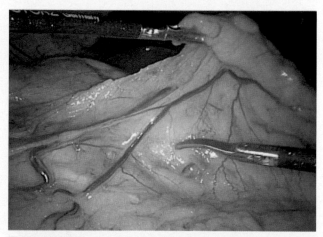

Figure 4H.2 The hepatic flexure is visualized and the ligament is divided with cautery, demonstrating an avascular plane.

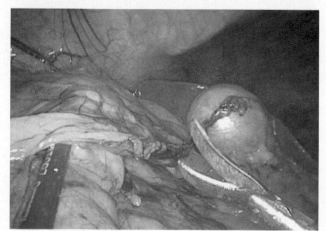

Figure 4H.3 As the hepatocolic ligament is divided, one enters the plane of prior dissection from the retroperitoneal mobilization of the ascending colon.

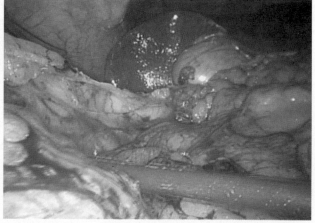

Figure 4H.4 The hepatic flexure is dissected off the pancreas and duodenum.

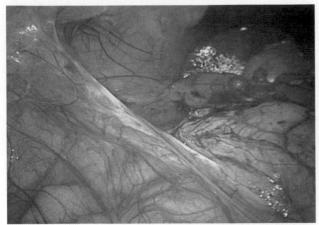

Figure 4H.5 The dissection is completed as the entire hepatic flexure and ascending colon are mobilized to the midline.

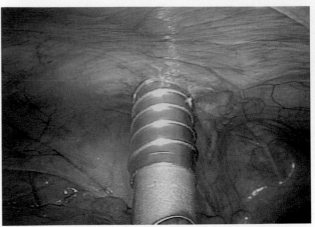

Figure 4I.1 The port is removed and a finger placed through the fascia to limit the air leak.

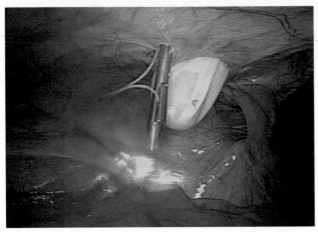

Figure 4I.2 A digit is placed through the port site to guide the end.

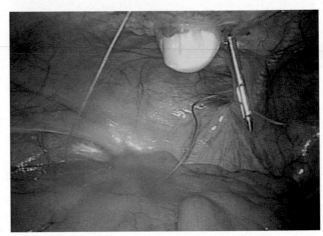

Figure 4I.3 The ENDO CLOSE is passed through the other side of the fascia and used to grasp the previously-inserted end of the ligature.

Operative Procedures

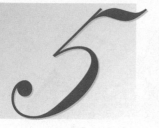

A | RIGHT HEMICOLECTOMY

KEY STEPS

1. Insertion of ports: 10-mm umbilical Hasson technique; 12-mm left iliac fossa; 5-mm left upper quadrant; 5-mm right iliac fossa (optional).

2. Patient rotated to the left and slightly Trendelenburg.

3. Laparoscopic assessment, and small bowel and omentum moved toward left upper quadrant.

4. Ileocolic pedicle defined and divided, protecting ureter and duodenum.

5. Hepatic flexure mobilized with superior approach.

6. Cecum retracted cranially and laterally for medial dissection of ascending colon.

7. Confirmation of full mobilization of right colon to midline.

8. Division of right branch of middle colic vessels.

9. Closure of ports >5 mm in size.

10. Umbilical incision and exteriorization of right colon.

11. Standard extracorporeal resection and anastomosis.

PATIENT POSITIONING

The patient is placed supine on the operating table, on a beanbag. After induction of general anesthesia and insertion of an oro-gastric tube and Foley catheter, the legs are placed in Dan Allen or Yellowfin stirrups (see Figure 5A.1). The arms are tucked at the patient's side and the beanbag is aspirated. The abdomen is prepared with antiseptic solution and draped routinely (see Chapter 4).

INSTRUMENT POSITIONING

The primary monitor is placed on the right side of the patient, up toward the patient's head. The secondary monitor is placed on the left side of the patient at the same level,

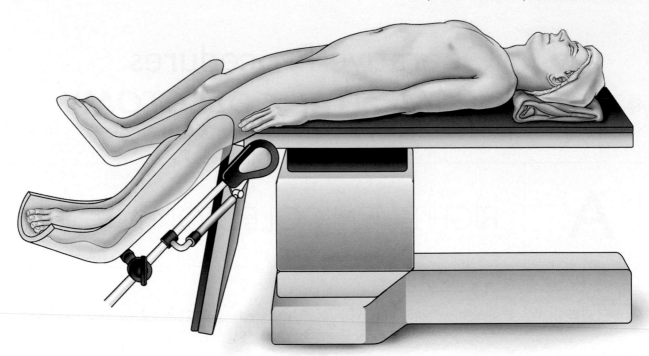

Figure 5A.1 The patient is positioned on the table in Dan Allen stirrups.

and is primarily for the assistant during the early phase of the surgery and port insertion (see Figure 5A.2). The operating nurse's instrument table is placed between the patient's legs. There should be sufficient space to allow the operating surgeon to move from either side of the patient to between the patient's legs, if necessary. The primary operating surgeon stands on the left side of the patient with the assistant standing on the patient's right, and moving to the left side, caudad to the surgeon, once ports have been inserted. A 0-degree camera lens is used.

UMBILICAL PORT INSERTION

This is performed using a modified Hasson approach (see Chapter 4). A vertical 1-cm subumbilical incision is made. This is deepened down to the linea alba, which is then grasped on each side of the midline using Kocher clamps. A scalpel (No. 15 blade) is used to open the fascia between the Kocher clamps and a Kelly forceps is used to open the peritoneum, bluntly. It is important to keep this opening small (<1 cm) to minimize air leaks. Having confirmed entry into the peritoneal cavity, a purse-string suture of 0 polyglycolic acid is placed around the subumbilical fascial defect (umbilical port site) and a Rommel tourniquet is applied. A 10-mm reusable port is inserted through this port site allowing the abdomen to be insufflated with CO_2 to a pressure of 12 mm Hg.

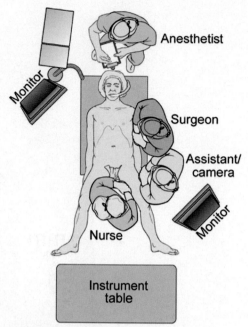

Figure 5A.2 Operating room setup for right side procedures.

LAPAROSCOPY AND INSERTION OF REMAINING PORTS

The camera is inserted into the abdomen and an initial laparoscopy is performed, carefully evaluating the liver, small bowel, and peritoneal surfaces. A 12-mm port is inserted through the left lower quadrant approximately 2 to 3 cm medial and superior to the anterior superior iliac spine (see Figure 5A.3). It is carefully inserted lateral to the inferior epigastric vessels, paying attention to keep the tract of the port going as perpendicular as possible through the abdominal wall. A 5-mm port is then inserted in the left upper quadrant at least a hand's breadth superior to the lower quadrant port. Particularly when teaching, a right lower quadrant 5-mm port is also inserted. Rarely, in the case of a difficult hepatic flexure, a 5-mm right upper quadrant port may also have to be inserted. Again, all of these remaining ports are kept lateral to the epigastric vessels. This may be ensured by diligence to anatomic port site selection and by using the laparoscope to transilluminate the abdominal wall before making the port site incision, to identify any obvious superficial vessels.

DEFINITIVE LAPAROSCOPIC SETUP

The assistant now moves to the patient's left side, standing caudad to the surgeon. The patient is rotated with the right side up and left side down, to approximately 15 to 20 degrees tilt, and often as far as the table can go. This helps to move the small bowel over to the left side of the abdomen. The patient is then placed in the Trendelenburg position. This again helps gravitational migration of the small bowel away from the operative field. The surgeon then inserts two atraumatic bowel clamps through the two left-sided abdominal ports. The greater omentum is reflected over the transverse colon so that

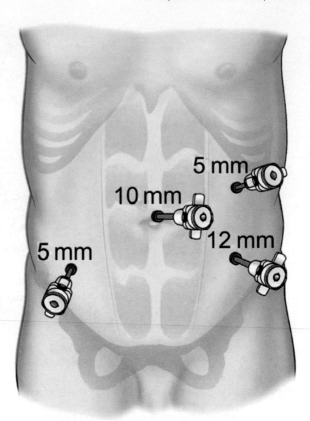

Figure 5A.3 Port setup for right side procedures.

it comes to lie on the stomach. If there is no space in the upper part of the abdomen, one must confirm that the orogastric tube is adequately decompressing the stomach. The small bowel is moved to the patient's left side, some remaining in the pelvis and upper abdomen, allowing visualization of the ileocolic pedicle (see Figure 5A.4). This may necessitate the use of the assistant's 5-mm atraumatic bowel clamp through the right lower quadrant to tent the ileal mesentery, medially and cephalad.

DEFINING AND DIVIDING THE ILEOCOLIC PEDICLE

A noncrushing bowel clamp is placed on the mesentery just at the ileocecal junction. This area is then stretched up toward the right lower quadrant port, stretching the vessel and also lifting it up from the retroperitoneum. In almost all cases, this demonstrates a sulcus between the medial side of the ileocolic pedicle and the retroperitoneum. Cautery is used to open the peritoneum along this line. Blunt dissection is then used to lift the vessel away from the retroperitoneum, opening the plane cranially up to the origin of the ileocolic artery from the superior mesenteric artery (see Figures 5A.5 and 5A.6). Cautery is then used to open a window in the peritoneum lateral to the vessel. Care is taken to make sure that the plane of dissection is anterior to the congenital layer of peritoneum, lying over the retroperitoneum, duodenum, and ureter. As long as this layer is preserved and the dissection is anterior to the duodenum, then we do not, as a routine, display the right ureter. The vessel is then divided (see Figure 5A.7). A clamp is placed on the origin of the vessel to control it if clips or other energy sources do not adequately control the vessel. When possible, clips are used to divide the vessel in an effort to minimize costs. Laparoscopic staplers or other energy sources may also be used. Having divided the vessel, the plane between the ascending colon mesentery and the retroperitoneum is developed laterally, out to the lateral attachment of the colon, and superiorly, dissecting the bowel off the anterior surface of the duodenum and pancreas (see Figures 5A.8–5A.10).

MOBILIZATION OF THE HEPATIC FLEXURE

The assistant now grasps the ascending colon with the atraumatic bowel clamp and draws it inferiorly. The surgeon grasps the proximal transverse colon with the atraumatic bowel clamp in his left hand and exerts traction on the ascending colon, medially and inferiorly. This maneuver puts the hepatic flexure under tension and permits division of the gastrocolic ligament using the scissors and cautery in the surgeon's right hand (see Figure 5A.11). The surgeon continues to progress along this mobilization plane to draw the hepatic flexure, inferiorly and medially (see Figure 5A.12). Care must be taken to avoid injury to the gallbladder and the second part of the duodenum as they are encountered while the hepatic flexure is mobilized. As the gastrocolic ligament is divided, the direction of traction on the transverse colon changes more to elevation and medial traction on the transverse colon by the assistant, and medial traction on the proximal colon by the surgeon (see Figure 5A.13).

As this dissection continues, the area of prior retroperitoneal dissection after division of the ileocolic pedicle becomes apparent. Once this area has been entered, it becomes clear that the only remaining attachment is the lateral peritoneal attachment along the ascending colon. This area, the white line of Toldt, is divided using cautery (see Figure 5A.14). This line is divided right down to the base of the cecum, and it may even be possible to completely mobilize the appendix and the base of the cecum to the midline from this direction. The colon is then dissected completely free from the underlying duodenum and retroperitoneum, and reflected entirely to the midline. This completes the hepatic flexure mobilization using the lateral-to-medial approach.

Mobilization of the hepatic flexure can be difficult. In patients who are very obese it can be hard to complete the ascending colon mobilization to the level of the hepatic flexure. In these cases, the release of the hepatic flexure can sometimes be facilitated by turning the patient to an anti-Trendelenburg position. Mobilization can sometimes be facilitated by inserting an instrument in the right upper quadrant. This additional port may provide additional traction on the hepatic flexure. The surgeon may find it more comfortable to stand between the patient's legs and use the two inferiorly placed ports as the main dissection instruments.

Having mobilized the hepatic flexure, attention is turned to the transverse colon mesentery. The right branches of the middle colic vessels are defined and can be divided with clips or an energy source of choice. This will allow complete removal of the specimen at the conclusion of the procedure with easy reach of colon for an adequate resection and easy anastomosis.

MOBILIZATION OF THE ILEOCECAL JUNCTION

The patient is then placed more into the Trendelenburg position, and the small bowel is reflected superiorly. The base of the attachment between the small bowel and terminal ileal mesentery and retroperitoneum is then seen. The mesentery of the terminal ileum is then elevated to expose the junction of the visceral peritoneum and the retroperitoneum. Scissors and cautery are used to dissect the terminal ileum off the retroperitoneal structures. Usually, there is only a thin layer of peritoneum that remains that needs division (see Figure 5A.15). This line of dissection extends from the ileocecal junction toward the origin of the superior mesenteric artery. Having initially started this dissection with cautery, the more proximal aspect of the mobilization should be performed with scissors alone. This is to avoid injury to the third part of the duodenum, which begins to appear near the end of the dissection. The plane between the retroperitoneum and the terminal ileum is developed and the terminal ileum is reflected, medially and cephalad. The iliac vessels, right ureter, and gonadal vessels all remain under the parietal peritoneum. It is important to complete the medial dissection to the level of the duodenum to facilitate eventual delivery of the complete specimen at the end of the procedure (see Figure 5A.16). All this dissection is performed with the atraumatic bowel clamp in the surgeon's left hand and the scissors in the right. The assistant's atraumatic bowel clamp may be used to help elevate the terminal ileum while it is reflected superiorly.

Before extracting the specimen, the surgeon should grasp the right colon and draw it to the left side and make sure that it is now mobilized to be entirely a midline structure (see Figure 5A.17). In some cases, there are remnant areolar attachments that may be divided. It is essential that the root of the ileal mesentery is as mobile as possible to permit easy retraction of the small bowel through the midline incision. A final check on complete mobility of the entire specimen and hemostasis is made before extracting the specimen.

SPECIMEN EXTRACTION

The 12-mm port site is closed using the ENDO CLOSE instrument. The appendix or the cecum is now grasped firmly through the right lower quadrant port site with an atraumatic bowel clamp. The pneumoperitoneum is deflated through the ports. The subumbilical port is removed and this port site is extended into a 3 to 4 cm midline incision. This may be made larger, if necessary, to remove larger phlegmons or tumors. In cases with a polyp or cancer, a wound protector is inserted to reduce the risk of tumor implantation in the wound.

The right colon is then exteriorized (see Figure 5A.18). The distal small bowel is assessed and the small bowel mesentery is divided extracorporeally using 0 polyglycolate suture ties for hemostasis. In cases of a bulky ileal mesentery, suture ligation of the mesentery may be used. The bowel is divided with a GIA 55 stapler and an Allis clamp is placed on the proximal end of the small bowel so that it is not lost back into the abdomen.

Attention is now turned to the area for division of the colon. The colonic mesentery is divided with cautery. Pulsatile mesenteric bleeding is confirmed and the vessel is ligated with 0 polyglycolate suture ties. Again, the colon is divided with the GIA 55. The specimen is now removed from the field and examined to confirm the pathologic findings, and the adequacy of proximal and distal margins. A side-to-side anastomosis is performed with the GIA 55 stapler, buttressing the crotch of the anastomosis with an interrupted 3/0 polyglycolate suture. The resulting opening from the GIA 55 stapler insertion site is then closed with a PI 55 stapler. The anastomosis is checked for hemostasis and returned to the abdomen.

The mesenteric window is not closed. The fascia is closed with interrupted figure-of-eight 1 polydioxanone sutures. The subcutaneous space is irrigated and the wounds are closed with subcuticular 4/0 polyglycolate sutures (see Figure 5A.19). The patient is woken up, extubated, and transferred to recovery to follow the standard postoperative care plan (see Chapter 3).

B | ILEOCECECTOMY

KEY STEPS

1. Insertion of ports: 10 mm umbilical Hasson technique; 5 mm left iliac fossa; 5 mm left upper quadrant; 5 mm right iliac fossa (optional).

2. Patient placed in Trendelenburg position and rotated to the left.

3. Reflection of small bowel and omentum cephalad.

4. Mobilize terminal ileum and cecum from retroperitoneum.

5. Lateral-to-medial mobilization of ascending colon.

6. Superior approach to hepatic flexure.

7. Extraction of terminal ileum and cecum.

8. Standard extracorporeal resection and anastomosis.

9. Assessment of entire small bowel to duodenojejunal flexure.

10. Examination of entire length of small bowel.

PATIENT POSITIONING

The patient is placed supine on the operating table, on a beanbag. After induction of general anesthesia and insertion of an oral gastric tube and Foley catheter, the legs are placed in Dan Allen or Yellowfin stirrups (see Figure 5B.1). The arms are tucked at the patient's side and the beanbag is aspirated. The abdomen is prepared with antiseptic solution and draped routinely (see Chapter 4).

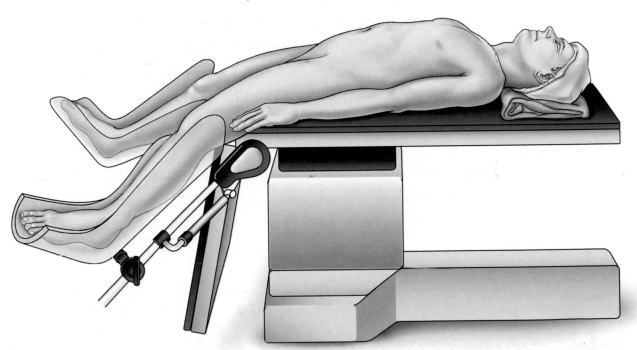

Figure 5B.1 The patient is positioned on the table in Dan Allen stirrups.

INSTRUMENT POSITIONING

The primary monitor is placed on the right side of the patient up toward the patient's head. The secondary monitor is placed on the left side of the patient at the same level, and is primarily for the assistant during the early phase of the surgery and port insertion (see Figure 5B.2). The operating nurse's instrument table is placed between the patient's legs. There should be sufficient space to allow the surgeon to move from either side of the patient to between the patient's legs, if necessary. The primary operating

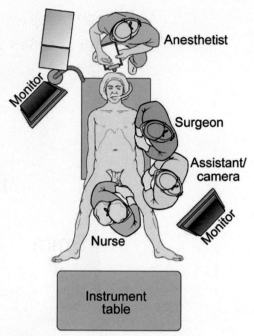

Figure 5B.2 Operating room setup for right side procedures.

surgeon stands on the left side of the patient with the assistant standing on the patient's right, and moving to the left side, caudad to the surgeon, once ports have been inserted. A 0-degree camera lens is used.

UMBILICAL PORT INSERTION

This is performed using a modified Hasson approach (see Chapter 4). A vertical 1-cm subumbilical incision is made. This is deepened down to the linea alba, which is then grasped on each side of the midline using Kocher clamps. A scalpel (No. 15 blade) is used to open the fascia between the Kocher clamps and a Kelly forceps is used to open the peritoneum bluntly. It is important to keep this opening small (<1 cm) to minimize air leaks. Having confirmed entry into the peritoneal cavity, a purse-string suture of 0 polyglycolic acid is placed around the subumbilical fascial defect (umbilical port site) and a Rommel tourniquet is applied. A 10-mm reusable port is inserted through this port site allowing the abdomen to be insufflated with CO_2 to a pressure of 12 mm Hg.

LAPAROSCOPY AND INSERTION OF REMAINING PORTS

The camera is inserted into the abdomen and an initial laparoscopy is performed, carefully evaluating the liver, small bowel, and peritoneal surfaces (see Figure 5B.3). A 5-mm port is inserted through the left lower quadrant approximately 2 to 3 cm medial and superior to the anterior superior iliac spine. This is carefully inserted lateral to the inferior epigastric vessels, paying attention to keep the tract of the port going as perpendicular as possible through the abdominal wall. A 5-mm port is then inserted in the left upper quadrant at least

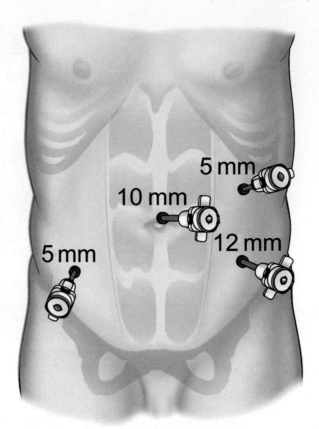

Figure 5B.3 Port setup for right side procedures.

a hand's breadth superior to the lower quadrant port. Particularly when teaching, a right lower quadrant 5-mm port is also inserted. Rarely, in the case of a difficult hepatic flexure, a 5-mm right upper quadrant port may also be needed to be inserted. Again, all these remaining ports are kept lateral to the epigastric vessels. This may be ensured by diligence to anatomical port site selection and using the laparoscope to transilluminate the abdominal wall before making the port site incision, to identify any obvious superficial vessels.

DEFINITIVE LAPARO-SCOPIC SETUP

The assistant now moves to the patient's left side, standing caudad to the surgeon. The patient is rotated with the right side up and left side down, to approximately 15 to 20 degrees tilt, and often as far as the table can go. This helps to move the small bowel over to the left side of the abdomen. The patient is then placed in the Trendelenburg position. This again helps gravitational migration of the small bowel away from the operative field. The surgeon then inserts two atraumatic bowel clamps through the two left-sided abdominal ports. The greater omentum is reflected over the transverse colon so that it comes to lie on the stomach. If there is no space in the upper part of the abdomen, one must confirm that the orogastric tube is adequately decompressing the stomach. Any remaining mobile small bowel is reflected from the pelvis into the upper abdomen. The terminal ileum is reflected cephalad to expose the fusion plane between the ileal mesentery and the parietal peritoneum covering the retroperitoneal structures. This may necessitate the use of the assistant's 5-mm atraumatic bowel clamp through the right lower quadrant to tent the ileal mesentery, medially and cephalad.

MOBILIZATION OF THE ILEOCECAL JUNCTION

Having tented up the mesentery of the terminal ileum to expose the junction of the visceral peritoneum and the retroperitoneum, scissors and cautery are used to dissect the terminal ileum off the retroperitoneal structures (see Figures 5B.4 and 5B.5). This line of dissection extends from the ileocecal junction toward the origin of the superior mesenteric artery. The focus of the dissection is now to mobilize the ileocecal junction from lateral to medial. The mobilization of the cecum should be completed before turning to the full mobilization of the terminal ileum. All the dissection is from lateral to medial and the dissection plane is continued under the terminal ileum, as it is reflected superiorly and medially. Having initially started this dissection with cautery, the more proximal aspect of the mobilization should be performed with scissors alone. This is to avoid injury to the third part of the duodenum, which begins to appear near the end of the dissection. The plane between the retroperitoneum and the terminal ileum is developed and the terminal ileum reflected, medially and cephalad. The terminal ileum may be quite bulky due to the underlying ileitis; however, this becomes easier as it is reflected from the fusion plane. The iliac vessels, right ureter, and gonadal vessels all remain under the parietal peritoneum and the dissection is carried medial to expose the duodenum (see Figure 5B.6). It is important to complete the medial dissection to the level of the duodenum to facilitate eventual delivery of the complete specimen at the end of the procedure. All this dissection is performed with the atraumatic bowel clamp in the surgeon's left hand and the scissors in the right. The assistant's atraumatic bowel clamp is used to help elevate the terminal ileum while it is reflected superiorly. Once the terminal ileum is mobilized sufficiently, the right paracolic attachments of the ascending colon may be displayed with traction of the ileocecal junction to permit lateral-to-medial mobilization of the ascending colon from the paracolic gutter. This line of dissection is carried superiorly as far as the hepatic flexure. Care must be taken not to inadvertently mobilize the duodenum or kidney, medially.

MOBILIZATION OF THE HEPATIC FLEXURE

Having divided the ascending colonic attachments, the assistant now grasps the transverse colon with the atraumatic bowel clamp and pushes it inferiorly. The surgeon grasps the distal ascending colon with the atraumatic bowel clamp in his right hand and exerts traction on the ascending colon, medially and inferiorly (see Figure 5B.7). This maneuver puts the hepatic flexure under tension and permits division of the gastrocolic ligament, using scissors and cautery. The surgeon continues to progress along this mobilization plane to draw the hepatic flexure inferiorly and medially (see Figure 5B.8). Care must be taken to avoid injury to the gallbladder and the second part of the duodenum as they are encountered while the hepatic flexure is mobilized. As the gastrocolic ligament is divided, the direction of traction on the transverse colon changes more to elevation and medial traction on the transverse colon by the assistant, and medial traction on the proximal colon by the surgeon. The colon is then dissected completely free from the underlying duodenum and reflected toward the midline (see Figures 5B.9 and 5B.10). This completes the hepatic flexure mobilization using the lateral-to-medial approach.

Mobilization of the hepatic flexure can be difficult. In patients who are very obese, it can be hard to complete the ascending colon mobilization to the level of the hepatic flexure. In these cases, the release of the hepatic flexure can sometimes be facilitated by turning the patient to an anti-Trendelenburg position. Mobilization can sometimes be facilitated by inserting an instrument in the right upper quadrant. This additional port may provide additional traction on the hepatic flexure. The surgeon may find it more comfortable to stand between the patient's legs and use the two inferiorly placed ports as the main dissection instruments.

Before extracting the specimen, the surgeon should revisit the base of the ileal mesentery. This may have remnant attachments that may be divided. It is essential that the root of the ileal mesentery is as mobile as possible to permit easy retraction of the small bowel through the midline incision. A final check on complete mobility of the entire specimen and hemostasis is made before extracting the specimen.

SPECIMEN EXTRACTION

The appendix or the cecum is now grasped firmly through the right lower quadrant port site with an atraumatic bowel clamp. The pneumoperitoneum is deflated through the ports. The subumbilical port is removed and this port site is extended into a 3 to 4 cm midline incision. This may be made larger, if necessary, to remove larger phlegmons. The colon and terminal ileum are then exteriorized through this site (see Figure 5B.11). The distal small bowel is assessed and the small bowel mesentery is divided extracorporeally using 0 polygalactin suture ties for hemostasis. In cases of a bulky ileal mesentery, suture ligation of the mesentery may be used. The bowel is divided with a GIA 55 stapler and an Allis clamp is placed on the proximal end of the small bowel so that it is not lost back into the abdomen. For Crohn's disease, a 2-cm margin of palpably normal bowel and mesentery is adequate.

Attention is now turned to the area for division of the colon. The colonic mesentery is divided with cautery. Pulsatile mesenteric bleeding is confirmed and the vessel is ligated with 0 polyglycolate suture ties. Again, the colon is divided with the GIA 55. The specimen is now removed from the field and examined to confirm the pathologic findings, and the adequacy of proximal and distal margins. A side-to-side anastomosis is performed with the GIA 55 stapler, buttressing the crotch of the anastomosis with an interrupted 3/0 polyglycolate suture. The resulting opening from the GIA 55 stapler insertion site is then closed with a PI 55 stapler. The anastomosis is checked for hemostasis and returned to the abdomen.

The small bowel may be exteriorized completely through the midline incision. This allows the surgeon to completely assess the small bowel for further evidence of Crohn's disease. Care must be taken while applying traction on the small bowel when exteriorizing it. In many cases, the anastomosis must be returned to the abdomen and the small bowel can then be run sequentially. The most proximal aspect of the small bowel to be reached is the paraduodenal fossa. These may be easily palpated with an educated digit, thereby formally identifying the duodenojejunal flexure (see Figure 5B.12). Any areas of obvious Crohn's enteritis may then be effectively treated at the surgeon's discretion. In cases where further resection or strictureplasty is required, it is advisable to return any excess exteriorized bowel into the abdomen to minimize traction on the superior mesenteric artery and avoid potential ischemia.

The mesenteric window is not closed. The fascia is closed with interrupted figure-of-eight I polydioxanone sutures. The subcutaneous space is irrigated and the wounds are closed with subcuticular 4/0 polyglycolate sutures. The patient is woken up, extubated, and transferred to recovery to follow the standard postoperative care plan (see Chapter 3).

C | SIGMOID COLECTOMY

 KEY STEPS

1. Insertion of ports: 10-mm umbilical Hasson technique; 12-mm right iliac fossa; 5-mm right upper quadrant; 5-mm left iliac fossa (optional).

2. Patient rotated to the right and slightly Trendelenburg.

3. Laparoscopic assessment, and small bowel and omentum moved toward right and upper quadrants.

4. Inferior mesenteric pedicle defined and divided, protecting ureter and presacral autonomic nerves.

5. Retroperitoneal mobilization of descending colon mesentery.

6. Division of lateral attachments of sigmoid and descending colon to splenic flexure.

7. Mobilization of rectosigmoid junction and choice of area for transection.

8. Transection of upper rectum and mesorectum.

9. Exteriorization and resection of sigmoid colon through left lower quadrant incision.

10. Reinsufflation and anastomosis.

11. Port closure.

PATIENT POSITIONING

The patient is placed supine on the operating table, on a beanbag. After induction of general anesthesia and insertion of an oral gastric tube and Foley catheter, the legs are placed in Dan Allen or Yellowfin stirrups (see Figure 5C.1). The arms are tucked at the patient's side and the beanbag is aspirated. The abdomen is prepared with antiseptic solution and draped routinely (see Chapter 4).

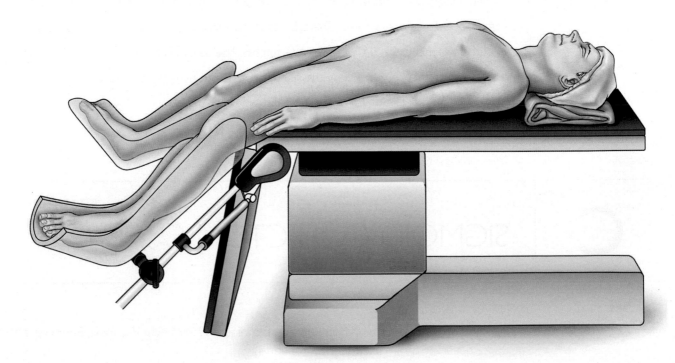

Figure 5C.1 The patient is positioned on the table in Dan Allen stirrups.

INSTRUMENT POSITIONING

The primary monitor is placed on the left side of the patient up toward his/her feet, at approximately the level of the hip. The secondary monitor is placed on the right side of the patient at the shoulder level, and is primarily for the assistant during the early phase of the surgery and port insertion (see Figure 5C.2). The operating nurse's instrument table is placed between the patient's legs. There should be sufficient space to allow the surgeon to move from either side of the patient to between the patient's legs, if necessary. The primary operating surgeon stands on the right side of the patient at the level of the patient's hip, with the assistant standing on the patient's left. The assistant moves to the right side at the level of the patient's shoulder, once the ports have been inserted. If a second assistant is available, he/she stays on the patient's left side. A 0-degree camera lens is used.

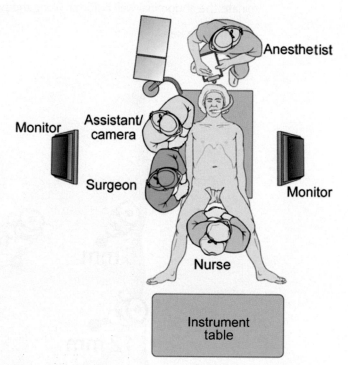

Figure 5C.2 Operating room setup for sigmoid procedures.

UMBILICAL PORT INSERTION

This is performed using a modified Hasson approach (see Chapter 4). A vertical 1-cm subumbilical incision is made. This is deepened down to the linea alba, which is then grasped on each side of the midline using Kocher clamps. A scalpel (No. 15 blade) is used to open the fascia between the Kocher clamps and a Kelly forceps is used to open the peritoneum, bluntly. It is important to keep this opening small (<1 cm) to minimize air leaks. Having confirmed entry into the peritoneal cavity, a purse-string suture of 0 polyglycolic acid is placed around the subumbilical fascial defect (umbilical port site) and a Rommel tourniquet is applied. A 10-mm reusable port is inserted through this port site allowing the abdomen to be insufflated with CO_2 to a pressure of 12 mm Hg.

LAPAROSCOPY AND INSERTION OF REMAINING PORTS

The camera is inserted into the abdomen and an initial laparoscopy performed, carefully evaluating the liver, small bowel, and peritoneal surfaces. A 12-mm port is inserted through the right lower quadrant approximately 2 to 3 cm medial and superior to the anterior superior iliac spine (see Figure 5C.3). It is carefully inserted lateral to the inferior epigastric vessels, paying attention to keep the tract of the port going as perpendicular as possible through the abdominal wall. A 5-mm port is then inserted in the right upper quadrant at least a hand's breadth superior to the lower quadrant port. Particularly when teaching, a left lower quadrant 5-mm port is also inserted. Rarely, in the case of a difficult splenic flexure, a 5-mm right upper quadrant port may also need to be inserted. Again, all of these remaining ports are kept lateral to the epigastric vessels. This may be ensured by diligence to anatomic port site selection and by using the laparoscope to transilluminate the abdominal wall before making the port site incision to identify any obvious superficial vessels.

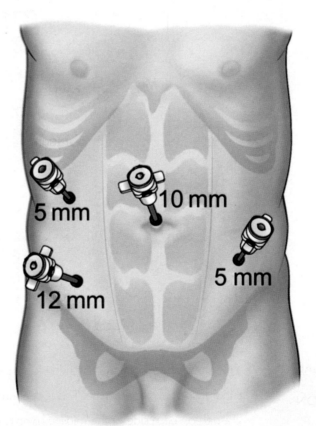

Figure 5C.3 Port setup for sigmoid procedures.

DEFINITIVE LAPARO-SCOPIC SETUP

The assistant now moves to the patient's right side, standing at shoulder level. The patient is rotated with the left side up and right side down, to approximately 15 to 20 degrees tilt, and often as far as the table can go. This helps to move the small bowel over to the right side of the abdomen. The patient is then placed in the Trendelenburg position. This again helps gravitational migration of the small bowel away from the operative field. The surgeon then inserts two atraumatic bowel clamps through the two left-sided abdominal ports. The greater omentum is reflected over the transverse colon so that it comes to lie on the stomach (see Figure 5C.4). If there is no space in the upper part of the abdomen, one must confirm that the orogastric tube is adequately decompressing the stomach. The small bowel is moved to the patient's right upper quadrant, allowing visualization of the inferior mesenteric pedicle. This may necessitate the use of the assistant's 5-mm atraumatic bowel clamp through the left lower quadrant to adequately tent up the sigmoid mesentery.

In patients with significant obesity or adhesions in the upper quadrants, it can be difficult to visualize the vascular pedicle. These adhesions may need to be lysed, or sometimes insertion of a left upper quadrant port allows use of another retractor to keep the small bowel out of the way. Such instruments are often left in place for some time, so we do not recommend clamping the intestine, but rather using a closed instrument to gently push a loop of intestine out of the way, and, if necessary, come back and check the field regularly.

DEFINING AND DIVIDING THE INFERIOR MESENTERIC PEDICLE

An atraumatic bowel clamp is placed on the rectosigmoid mesentery at the level of the sacral promontory, approximately half way between the bowel wall and the promontory itself. This area is then stretched up toward the left lower quadrant port, stretching the inferior mesenteric vessels away from the retroperitoneum (see Figure 5C.5). In most cases, this demonstrates a groove between the right or medial side of the inferior mesenteric pedicle and the retroperitoneum. Cautery is used to open the peritoneum along this line, opening the plane cranially up to the origin of the inferior mesenteric artery, and caudally past the sacral promontory (see Figure 5C.6). Blunt dissection is then used to lift the vessels away from the retroperitoneum and presacral autonomic nerves (see Figure 5C.7). The ureter is then looked for under the inferior mesenteric artery (see Figure 5C.8). If the ureter cannot be seen and the dissection is in the correct plane, the ureter should be just deep to the parietal peritoneum, and just medial to the gonadal vessels. Care must be taken not to dissect too deep and injure the iliac vessels.

If the ureter cannot be found, it has usually been elevated on the back of the inferior mesenteric pedicle, and one needs to stay very close to the vessel not only to find the ureter but also to protect the autonomic nerves. If the ureter still cannot be found, the dissection needs to come in a cranial direction, which is usually into clean tissue allowing it to be found. If this fails, a lateral approach can be performed (see subsequent text). This usually gives a fresh perspective to the tissues, and the ureter can often be found quite easily. In very rare cases, the ureter still may not be found. We do not routinely use ureteric stents, so the options at this stage include conversion to open surgery, or insertion of ureteric stents. We do not proceed if the ureter cannot be defined.

Cautery is then used to open a window in the peritoneum, lateral to the inferior mesenteric vessels (see Figure 5C.9). The vessel is then divided using a low ligation (distal to the left colic artery) for benign inflammatory disease (see Figure 5C.10), and a high ligation (above the left colic artery) for malignant disease. A clamp is placed on the origin of the vessel to control it if clips or other energy sources do not adequately control the vessel. In general for a left colectomy, a cartridge of the ENDO GIA stapler is used to divide the vessel. This helps minimize expenditure, as the stapler will anyway be required for division of the rectum. Laparoscopic clips or other energy sources may also be used.

Having divided the vessel, the plane between the descending colon mesentery and the retroperitoneum is developed laterally, out toward the lateral attachment of the colon, and superiorly, dissecting the bowel off the anterior surface of the Gerota's fascia up toward the splenic flexure (see Figure 5C.11) and the right side of the mesorectum is partially mobilized (see Figure 5C.12).

MOBILIZATION OF THE LATERAL ATTACH- MENTS OF THE RECTOSIG- MOID AND DESCENDING COLON

The surgeon now grasps the rectosigmoid junction with his left-hand instrument and draws it to the patient's right side (see Figure 5C.13). This allows the lateral attachments of the sigmoid colon to be seen and divided using cautery. Bruising from the prior retroperi- toneal mobilization of the colon can usually be seen in this area. Once this layer of peri- toneum has been opened, one immediately enters into the space opened by the retroperi- toneal dissection. Dissection now continues up along the white line of Toldt, toward the splenic flexure. As the dissection continues, the surgeon's left-hand instrument needs to be gradually moved up along the descending colon to keep the lateral attachments under tension. In this way, the lateral and any remaining posterior attachments are freed, making the left colon and sigmoid a midline structure (see Figure 5C.14). Elevating the descending colon and drawing it medially is useful, as this keeps small bowel loops out of the way of the dissecting instrument and facilitates the dissection.

For benign disease, we do not routinely mobilize the splenic flexure, but dissect up to this point. In some patients, particularly very obese or otherwise large patients, it is difficult to reach high enough through the right lower quadrant port. For this reason, the surgeon's right-hand instrument is moved to the left lower quadrant port site. This permits greater reach along the descending colon.

Attention is then turned to the lower attachments of the rectosigmoid, and cautery is used to open along the left lateral side of the upper mesorectum. The ureter is carefully observed and protected, and the bowel is mobilized to obtain a sufficient distal margin (see Figure 5C.15).

DIVISION OF THE UPPER RECTUM AND MESORECTUM

The assistant now grasps the rectosigmoid junction through the left lower quadrant port, and draws it up and out of the pelvis, and somewhat anteriorly (see Figure 5C.16). This gives the surgeon a nice view of the posterior surface of the mesorectum and the presacral space, and a decision can be made whether the dissection is adequate on the right side. Once the dissection is completed, the assistant draws the rectosigmoid out of the pelvis, without anterior displacement, giving the surgeon a good view of the right side of the mesorectum, and allowing a decision to be made about the distal margin of resection. If the surgery is being performed for malignancy, a flexible endoscope may be inserted to confirm that there is an adequate distal margin.

Cautery is used to open the peritoneum, perpendicular to the site to be transected. An atraumatic bowel grasper is then used to open a plane between the rectum and the mesorectum, by advancing the instrument between the two structures and separating the jaws in an anteroposterior direction (see Figure 5C.17). This reduces bleeding by minimizing avulsion of small vessels off the back of the mesorectum. Stretching the rectum up out of the pelvis, and drawing it somewhat to the patient's left allows the instrument to be passed through perpendicularly at the correct level.

An ENDO GIA stapler is then inserted through the right lower quadrant port and used to divide the rectum, and two firings are usually required (see Figure 5C.18). If one cartridge is adequate, it is usually because the patient has a small body habitus, or because one is up too far on the narrower sigmoid colon.

The assistant now grasps the divided proximal end of the rectum and draws it anteriorly and to the left. This tents up the mesorectum and displays it so that the surgeon can divide it. Our practice is usually to use monopolar or bipolar cautery, although clips or other energy sources can be used (see Figure 5C.19). Before dividing the final strand of the mesorectum, the distal end is carefully examined for hemostasis, as once the mesorectum is completely divided the rectum retracts deep down into the pelvis (see Figure 5C.20).

Before extracting the specimen, the surgeon should grasp the divided proximal end of the rectum and a final check on complete mobility of the entire specimen and hemostasis should be made (see Figure 5C.21).

SPECIMEN EXTRACTION

A 3 to 4 cm left lower quadrant muscle–splitting incision is then made, through the left lower quadrant port site. This may be made larger, if necessary, to remove larger phlegmons or tumors. In cases with a polyp or cancer, a wound protector is inserted to reduce the risk of tumor implantation in the wound.

The specimen is then exteriorized. The descending colon mesentery is divided extra-corporeally using 0 polyglycolate suture ties for hemostasis, and confirming the presence of pulsatile bleeding in the mesentery (see Figure 5C.22). The bowel is divided between noncrushing bowel clamps, and a Babcock clamp is placed on the proximal end of the colon so that it is not lost back into the abdomen. The specimen is examined for ade-quacy of margins. A size 0 polypropylene purse-string suture is inserted and the anvil of a size-29 circular stapler is inserted (see Figure 5C.23). The bowel is returned to the abdomen and the fascia is closed with layers of 1 polyglycolate.

ANASTOMOSIS

The abdomen is reinsufflated and the proximal colon is found. Adequacy of reach is then determined by placing the colon with anvil, into the pelvis (see Figure 5C.24). If it lies spontaneously, then anastomotic tension will normally be absent. If the colon keeps falling back into the abdomen, then further mobilization of the splenic flexure is required (see Chapter 4G). Orientation is confirmed by following the cut edge of the mesentery back to the retroperitoneum (see Figure 5C.25).

The circular stapler is then inserted into the rectum and carefully advanced up to the apex of the rectal stump. The anastomosis is closed and performed routinely and usually lies about one-third of the way down into the pelvis (see Figures 5C.26 and 5C.27). The "doughnuts" are examined for completeness. The colon is gently grasped at approximately the level of the sacral promontory and the pelvis is filled with irrigating fluid. The anastomosis is tested by distending the rectum with air, using a proctoscope or bulb syringe (see Figure 5C.28). Anastomotic tension is assessed by placing an instrument behind the mesentery, just above the sacral promontory, and elevating the colon away from the retroperitoneum.

Occasionally, it may be difficult to get the stapler to reach the apex of the rectal stump. The use of plenty of lubricant is important. Advancing the instrument with a rotating movement also helps it to slide by some mucosal folds. Great care must be taken if any instrument is used to hold the rectal stump, as it can very easily perforate the stump or leave a tear in the serosa.

In some cases it is not possible to get the stapler in position. Two options are available. One is to extrude the spike of the stapler on the anterior wall of the rectum and perform an end-to-side anastomosis. The second is to resect more rectum, going down to where the circular stapler has reached, using an extra cartridge of the ENDO GIA instrument. This permits a standard end-to-end anastomosis to be completed.

Hemostasis is confirmed and the abdomen is irrigated. The right lower quadrant port is closed with an ENDO CLOSE, and the remaining ports are removed. The purse-string suture, which had been placed at the umbilical port site, is tied to close the fascia at this site. The subcutaneous spaces are then irrigated, and the wounds are closed with subcuticular 4/0 polyglycolate sutures. The patient is woken up, extubated, and transferred to recovery to follow the standard postoperative care plan (see Chapter 3).

RECTAL SURGERY

D | LOW ANTERIOR RESECTION

KEY STEPS

1. Insertion of ports: 10-mm umbilical Hasson technique; 12-mm right iliac fossa; 5-mm right upper quadrant; 5-mm left upper quadrant; 5-mm left iliac fossa.

2. Patient rotated to the right and Trendelenburg.

3. Laparoscopic assessment, and small bowel and omentum moved toward right upper quadrant.

4. Inferior mesenteric artery pedicle identified and dissected. Left ureter identified and inferior mesenteric artery divided near origin.

5. Medial-to-lateral mobilization of left colon and division of inferior mesenteric vein.

6. Lateral paracolic mobilization of left colon toward splenic flexure.

7. Splenic flexure mobilization.

8. Rectal mobilization. Dissection behind rectum down presacral plane.

9. Division of peritoneal attachments on right and left side of rectum, and anterior mobilization beginning at peritoneal reflection.

10. Rectum stapled at pelvic floor and divided.

11. Extracorporeal resection and stapled coloanal anastomosis.

12. Formation of right iliac fossa trephine loop ileostomy.

13. Closure of ports >5 mm in size.

PATIENT POSITIONING

The patient is placed supine on the operating table, on a beanbag. After induction of general anesthesia and insertion of an orogastric tube and Foley catheter, the legs are placed in Dan Allen or Yellowfin stirrups (see Figure 5D.1). The arms are tucked at the patient's side and the beanbag is aspirated. The abdomen is prepared with antiseptic solution and draped routinely (see Chapter 4).

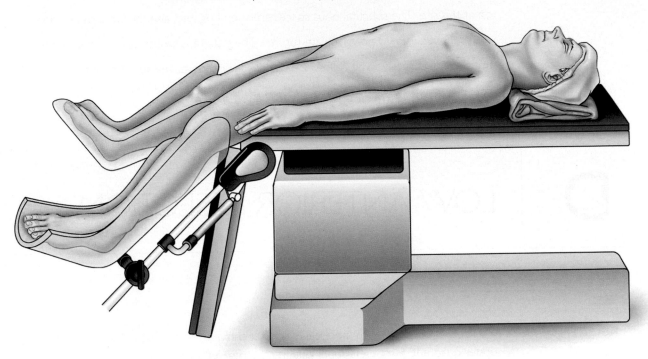

Figure 5D.1 The patient is positioned on the table in Dan Allen stirrups.

INSTRUMENT POSITIONING

The primary monitor is placed on the left side of the patient at approximately the level of the hip. The secondary monitor is placed on the right side of the patient at the same level, and is primarily for the assistant during the early phase of the surgery and port insertion (see Figure 5D.2). The operating nurse's instrument table is placed between the patient's legs. There should be sufficient space to allow the surgeon to move from either side of the patient to between the patient's legs, if necessary. The primary operating surgeon stands on the right side of the patient with the assistant standing on the patient's left, and moving to the right side, caudad to the surgeon, once ports have been inserted. A 0-degree camera lens is used.

UMBILICAL PORT INSERTION

This is performed using a modified Hasson approach (see Chapter 4). A vertical 1-cm subumbilical incision is made. This is deepened down to the linea alba, which is then grasped on each side of the midline using Kocher clamps. A scalpel (No. 15 blade) is used to open the fascia between the Kocher clamps and a Kelly forceps is used to open the peritoneum, bluntly. It is important to keep this opening small (<1 cm) to minimize

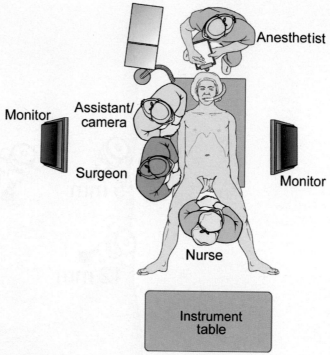

Figure 5D.2 Operating room setup for sigmoid procedures.

air leaks. Having confirmed entry into the peritoneal cavity, a purse-string suture of 0 polyglycolic acid is placed around the subumbilical fascial defect (umbilical port site) and a Rommel tourniquet is applied. A 10-mm reusable port is inserted through this port site allowing the abdomen to be insufflated with CO_2 to a pressure of 12 mm Hg.

LAPAROSCOPY AND INSERTION OF REMAINING PORTS

The camera is inserted into the abdomen and an initial laparoscopy is performed, carefully evaluating the liver, small bowel, and peritoneal surfaces. A 12-mm port is inserted in the right lower quadrant approximately 2 to 3 cm medial and superior to the anterior superior iliac spine (see Figure 5D.3). It is carefully inserted lateral to the inferior epigastric vessels, paying attention to keep the tract of the port going as perpendicular as possible through the abdominal wall. A 5-mm port is then inserted in the right upper quadrant at least a hand's breadth superior to the lower quadrant port. A left lower quadrant 5-mm port is inserted. A 5-mm left upper quadrant port is also inserted to aid splenic flexure mobilization. Again, all of these remaining ports are kept lateral to the epigastric vessels. This may be ensured by diligence to anatomic port site selection and using the laparoscope to transilluminate the abdominal wall before making the port site incision to identify any obvious superficial vessels.

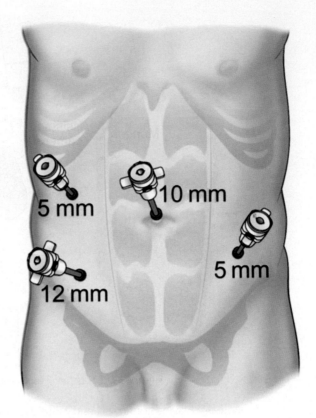

Figure 5D.3 Port setup for sigmoid procedures.

DEFINITIVE LAPARO-SCOPIC SETUP

The assistant now moves to the patient's left side, standing caudad to the surgeon. The patient is rotated with the left side up and right side down, to approximately 15 to 20 degrees tilt, and often as far as the table can go. This helps to move the small bowel over to the right side of the abdomen. The patient is then placed in the Trendelenburg position. This again helps gravitational migration of the small bowel away from the operative field. The surgeon then inserts two atraumatic bowel clamps through the two right-sided abdominal ports. The greater omentum is reflected over the transverse colon so that it comes to lie on the stomach. If there is no space in the upper part of the abdomen, one must confirm that the orogastric tube is adequately decompressing the stomach. The small bowel is moved to the patient's right side allowing visualization of the medial aspect of the rectosigmoid mesentery. This may necessitate the use of the assistant's 5-mm atraumatic bowel clamp through the left lower quadrant to tent the sigmoid mesentery cephalad.

DEFINING AND DIVIDING THE INFERIOR MESENTERIC PEDICLE

An atraumatic bowel clamp is placed on the rectosigmoid mesentery at the level of the sacral promontory, approximately half way between the bowel wall and the promontory itself. This area is then stretched up toward the left lower quadrant port, stretching the inferior mesenteric vessels away from the retroperitoneum. In most cases this demonstrates a groove between the right or medial side of the inferior mesenteric pedicle and the retroperitoneum. Cautery is used to open the peritoneum along this line, opening the plane cranially up to the origin of the inferior mesenteric artery, and caudally past the sacral promontory. Blunt dissection is then used to lift the vessels away from the retroperitoneum and presacral autonomic nerves (see Figure 5D.4). The ureter is then looked for under the inferior mesenteric artery. If the ureter cannot be seen, and the dissection is in the correct plane, the ureter should be just deep to the parietal peritoneum, and just medial to the gonadal vessels. Care must be taken not to dissect too deep and injure the iliac vessels.

If the ureter cannot be found, it has usually been elevated on the back of the inferior mesenteric pedicle, and one needs to stay very close to the vessel not only to find the ureter but also to protect the autonomic nerves. If the ureter still cannot be found, the dissection needs to come in a cranial direction, which is usually into clean tissue allowing it to be found. If this fails, a lateral approach can be performed (see subsequent text). This usually gives a fresh perspective to the tissues, and the ureter can often be found quite easily. In very rare cases, the ureter still may not be found. We do not use ureteric stents as a routine, so the options at this stage include conversion to open surgery, or insertion of ureteric stents. We do not proceed if the ureter cannot be defined. The dissection is continued up to the origin of the inferior mesenteric artery, which is carefully defined and divided using a high ligation, above the left colic artery (see Figure 5D.5). A clamp is placed on the origin of the vessel to control it if clips or other energy sources do not adequately control the vessel. In general for a left colectomy, a cartridge of the ENDO GIA stapler is used to divide the vessel (see Figure 5D.6). This helps minimize expenditure, as the stapler will anyway be required for division of the rectum. Laparoscopic clips or other energy sources may also be used for the vessel. The inferior mesenteric vein can also be divided, and this can frequently be achieved with the same stapler cartridge as is being used for the artery (see Figure 5D.7).

Having divided the vessels at the origin of the artery, the plane between the descending colon mesentery and the retroperitoneum is developed laterally, out toward the lateral attachment of the colon, and superiorly, dissecting the bowel off the anterior surface of the Gerota's fascia up toward the splenic flexure. This makes the inferior vein quite obvious and this vessel can also be divided just inferior to the pancreas. This allows increased reach for a coloanal anastomosis with or without neorectal reservoir (see Figure 5D.8).

MOBILIZATION OF THE LATERAL ATTACH- MENTS OF THE RECTOSIG- MOID AND DESCENDING COLON

The surgeon now grasps the rectosigmoid junction with his left-hand instrument and draws it to the patient's right side. This allows the lateral attachments of the sigmoid colon to be seen and divided using cautery. Bruising from the prior retroperitoneal mobilization of the colon can usually be seen in this area. Once this layer of peritoneum has been opened, one immediately enters into the space opened by the retroperitoneal dissection. Dissection now continues up along the white line of Toldt, toward the splenic flexure. As the dissection continues, the surgeon's left-hand instrument needs to be gradually moved up along the descending colon to keep the lateral attachments under tension. In this way, the lateral and any remaining posterior attachments are freed, making the left colon and sigmoid a midline structure. Elevating the descending colon and drawing it medially is useful, as this keeps small bowel loops out of the way of the dissecting instrument and facilitates the dissection. In some patients, particularly very obese or otherwise large patients, it is difficult to reach high enough through the right lower quadrant port. For this reason, the surgeon's right-hand instrument is moved to the left lower quadrant port site. This permits greater reach along the descending colon.

MOBILIZATION OF THE SPLENIC FLEXURE

Complete lateral mobilization of the left colon up to the splenic flexure is performed as an initial step. The descending colon is pulled medially using an atraumatic bowel clamp in the right lower quadrant port and the scissors are placed in the left iliac fossa port. A 5-mm left upper quadrant port may be necessary, particularly in those with a very high splenic flexure, or in very tall or obese individuals. The lateral attachments of the left colon are divided and the colon is dissected off the Gerota's fascia over the left kidney (see Chapter 4G).

Once the lateral attachments of the colon have been freed, it is necessary to move medially and enter the lesser sac. Some surgeons prefer to perform this as an initial step before lateral mobilization. To enter the lesser sac, the patient is tilted to a slight reverse Trendelenburg position. An atraumatic bowel clamp is inserted through the right upper quadrant port. If the left upper quadrant port is available this is also used. The assistant holds up the greater omentum, toward its left side, like a cape. The surgeon grasps the transverse colon toward the left side using a grasper in the right lower quadrant port to aid identification of the avascular plane between the greater omentum and the transverse mesocolon. Diathermy scissors are used through the left lower quadrant port to dissect this plane and enter the lesser sac. The surgeon usually moves to stand between the patient's legs for this part of the procedure. This dissection is continued toward the splenic flexure.

Following separation of the omentum off the left side of the transverse colon, connection to the lateral dissection allows the splenic flexure to be fully mobilized. The colon at the flexure is retracted caudally and medially, and any remaining restraining attachments are divided.

RECTAL MOBILIZATION

The patient is returned to the Trendelenburg position, and the small bowel is reflected cranially. Atraumatic bowel clamps inserted through the left-sided ports are used to elevate the rectosigmoid colon out of the pelvis and away from the retroperitoneum and sacral promontory, to enable entry into the presacral space. The posterior aspect of the mesorectum can be identified and the mesorectal plane dissected with diathermy, preserving the hypogastric nerves as they pass down into the pelvis, anterior to the sacrum (see Figure 5D.9). Dissection continues down the presacral space in this avascular plane toward the pelvic floor (see Figure 5D.10).

Attention is now switched to the peritoneum on the right side of the rectum. This is divided to the level of the seminal vesicles or rectovaginal septum (see Figure 5D.11). This is repeated on the peritoneum on the left side of the rectum. This facilitates further posterior dissection along the back of the mesorectum to the pelvic floor, to a level inferior to the lower edge of the mesorectum, just posterior to the anal canal. For a low anterior resection, it is necessary to perform a total mesorectal excision and hence the rectum must be dissected down to the muscle tube of the rectum below the inferior extent of the mesorectum. In many cases, particularly in those who are obese or men with a narrow pelvis, some or all of the anterior and lateral dissection must be completed to get adequate visualization, to complete the posterior dissection (see Figure 5D.12).

An atraumatic bowel clamp through the left iliac fossa port is used to retract the peritoneum anterior to the rectum forward. The peritoneal dissection is continued from the free edge of the lateral peritoneal dissection, anteriorly (see Figure 5D.13). Lateral dissection is continued on both sides of the rectum and is extended anterior to the rectum, posterior to Denonvillier's fascia, separating the posterior vaginal wall from the anterior wall of the rectum or down to the level of the prostate in men. The difficulty of dissection will vary depending on the body habitus of the patient, the diameter of the pelvis, and the size of the tumor. Occasionally, rectal mobilization can be very difficult to perform laparoscopically. In some cases, it may need to be completed in an open manner through a small Pfannenstiel incision (see Figure 5D.14).

RECTAL DIVISION

The lower rectum may be divided with a stapler either laparoscopically or by open surgery, depending on the ease of access related to the size of the pelvis. A reticulating endoscopic stapler may be used laparoscopically to divide the muscle tube of the rectum below the level of the mesorectum. The stapler is inserted through the right lower quadrant incision, and two firings of the stapler are usually required to divide the rectum (see Figures 5D.15 and 5D.16). There is no residual mesorectum to divide at this level. Digital examination is performed to confirm the location of the distal staple line, and if there is any doubt about adequacy of the distal margin, a rigid proctoscopy is performed.

It is sometimes impossible to divide the rectum laparoscopically as the angulation of the endovascular stapler is limited to 45 degrees, necessitating open division of the rectum. In some patients, getting an assistant to push up on the perineum with their hand may lift the pelvic floor enough to get the first cartridge of the stapler low enough. In some cases, placing a suprapubic port allows easier access with the stapler to allow division of the rectum.

Some patients are either too obese or have a very narrow pelvis or a long anal canal, and the stapler cannot be passed low enough. Two options exist. One is to perform a transanal intersphincteric dissection, remove the specimen, and then perform a hand-sewn coloanal anastomosis. The second is to perform a short Pfannenstiel incision, which allows a linear 30-mm stapler to be positioned and the rectum divided.

SPECIMEN EXTRACTION AND ANASTOMOSIS

The specimen can be extracted either through a Pfannenstiel incision or a left iliac fossa incision; in both incisions, a wound protector is used in cases with a polyp or cancer to reduce the risk of tumor implantation in the wound. The left colon mesentery is divided with cautery. The left colon is divided and the specimen is removed (see Figure 5D.17).

Pulsatile mesenteric bleeding is confirmed and the vessels ligated with 0 polyglycolate suture ties. Depending on the preference of the operating surgeon, a colonic pouch or coloplasty may be performed. A 2/0 Prolene purse-string suture is inserted into the distal end of the left colon or pouch, the anvil of a circular stapling gun inserted, and the purse-string suture is tied tightly. If a Pfannenstiel incision has been made, the coloanal anastomosis can be performed under direct vision and open manipulation following insertion of a circular stapling gun into the rectal stump. If a left iliac fossa incision has been used, the colon is returned to the abdomen and the incision closed, the pneumoperitoneum recreated, and the anastomosis is formed laparoscopically. The anastomosis can be leak-tested by filling the pelvis with saline and inflating the neorectum using a proctoscope or bulb syringe.

A defunctioning loop ileostomy can be performed either as open surgery or laparoscopically (see Chapter 5L), again depending on the extraction site used previously.

PORT SITE CLOSURE

The right iliac fossa 12-mm port site is closed using an ENDO CLOSE (see Chapter 41).

The umbilical port site is closed using the previously inserted purse-string suture.

E | ABDOMINOPERINEAL RESECTION 🪩

KEY STEPS

1. Insertion of ports: 10-mm umbilical Hasson technique; 12-mm right iliac fossa; 5-mm left iliac fossa; 5-mm right upper quadrant.

2. Patient rotated to the right and Trendelenburg position.

3. Laparoscopic assessment, and small bowel and omentum moved toward right upper quadrant.

4. Inferior mesenteric artery pedicle identified and dissected. Left ureter identified and inferior mesenteric artery divided near origin.

5. Medial-to-lateral mobilization of left colon.

6. Division of left colon mesentery and left colon proximal to inferior mesenteric artery.

7. Rectal mobilization. Dissection behind rectum down presacral plane.

8. Rectal mobilization to pelvic floor.

9. Formation of trephine end colostomy in left iliac fossa.

10. Open perineal dissection, completion of rectal resection, and removal of specimen through perineum. Closure of perineal wound.

11. Closure of ports >5 mm size.

PATIENT POSITIONING

The patient is placed supine on the operating table on a beanbag. After induction of general anesthesia and insertion of an orogastric tube and Foley catheter, the legs are placed in Dan Allen or Yellowfin stirrups (see Figure 5E.1). The arms are tucked at the patient's side and the beanbag is aspirated. The abdomen is prepared with antiseptic solution and draped routinely (see Chapter 4).

INSTRUMENT POSITIONING

The primary monitor is placed on the left side of the patient up toward the patient's feet. The secondary monitor is placed on the right side of the patient at the same level, and

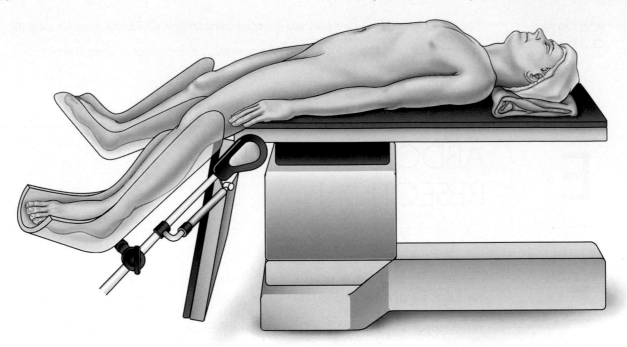

Figure 5E.1 The patient is positioned on the table in Dan Allen stirrups.

is primarily for the assistant during the early phase of the surgery and port insertion (see Figure 5E.2). The operating nurse's instrument table is placed between the patient's legs. There should be sufficient space to allow the surgeon to move from either side of the patient to between the patient's legs, if necessary. The primary operating surgeon stands on the right side of the patient with the assistant standing on the patient's left, and moving to the right side, caudad to the surgeon, once ports have been inserted. A 0-degree camera lens is used.

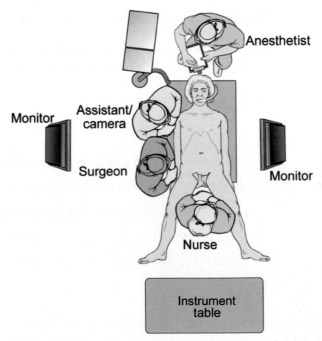

Figure 5E.2 Operating room setup for sigmoid procedures.

UMBILICAL PORT INSERTION

This is performed using a modified Hasson approach (see Chapter 4). A vertical 1-cm subumbilical incision is made. This is deepened down to the linea alba, which is then grasped on each side of the midline using Kocher clamps. A scalpel (No. 15 blade) is used to open the fascia between the Kocher clamps and a Kelly forceps is used to open the peritoneum bluntly. It is important to keep this opening small (<1 cm) to minimize air leaks. Having confirmed entry into the peritoneal cavity, a purse-string suture of 0 polyglycolic acid is placed around the subumbilical fascial defect (umbilical port site) and a Rommel tourniquet is applied. A 10-mm reusable port is inserted through this port site allowing the abdomen to be insufflated with CO_2 to a pressure of 12 mm Hg.

LAPAROSCOPY AND INSERTION OF REMAINING PORTS

The camera is inserted into the abdomen and an initial laparoscopy is performed, carefully evaluating the liver, small bowel, and peritoneal surfaces. A 12-mm port is inserted in the right lower quadrant approximately 2–3 cm medial and superior to the anterior superior iliac spine (see Figure 5E.3). This is carefully inserted lateral to the inferior epigastric vessels, paying attention to keep the tract of the port going as perpendicular as possible through the abdominal wall. A 5-mm port is then inserted in the right upper quadrant at least a hand's breadth superior to the lower quadrant port. A left lower

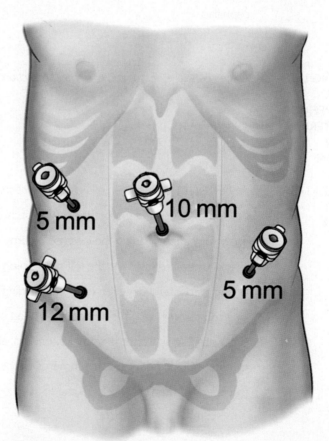

Figure 5E.3 Port setup for sigmoid procedures.

quadrant 5-mm port is also inserted. Again, all of these remaining ports are kept lateral to the epigastric vessels. This may be ensured by diligence to anatomic port site selection and using the laparoscope to transilluminate the abdominal wall before making the port site incision to identify any obvious superficial vessels.

DEFINITIVE LAPARO-SCOPIC SETUP

The assistant now moves to the patient's left side, standing caudad to the surgeon. The patient is rotated with the left side up and right side down, to approximately 15 to 20 degrees tilt, and often as far as the table can go. This helps to move the small bowel over to the right side of the abdomen. The patient is then placed in the Trendelenburg position. This again helps gravitational migration of the small bowel away from the operative field. The surgeon then inserts two atraumatic bowel clamps through the two right-sided abdominal ports. The greater omentum is reflected over the transverse colon so that it comes to lie on the stomach. If there is no space in the upper part of the abdomen, one must confirm that the orogastric tube is adequately decompressing the stomach. The small bowel is moved to the patient's right side allowing visualization of the medial aspect of the rectosigmoid mesentery pedicle. This may necessitate the use of the assistant's 5-mm atraumatic bowel clamp through the left lower quadrant to tent the sigmoid mesentery cephalad.

DEFINING LEFT URETER AND INFERIOR MESENTERIC ARTERY DIVISION

As per definitive description of sigmoid resection. (see Chapter 5C)

MOBILIZATION OF LEFT COLON

As per definitive description of sigmoid resection. (see Chapter 5C)

Complete mobilization of the left colon is not required. Adequate mobilization must allow formation of a left iliac fossa colostomy without tension. Following division of the inferior mesenteric artery, the left mesocolon is separated from the retroperitoneum in a medial-to-lateral direction using a spreading movement. An atraumatic bowel clamp inserted through a right-sided port is placed under the left colonic mesentery, which is elevated away from the retroperitoneum, and using a scissors inserted through the other right-sided port, the attachments to the retroperitoneum are swept down, until the lateral abdominal wall is reached.

DIVISION OF THE LEFT COLON

The mesentery of the left colon is divided from the free edge, cranial to the previously divided inferior mesenteric artery, toward the left sigmoid colon. The mesentery can be divided with diathermy and the marginal artery can be clipped and then divided. Alternatively, an energy source such as a LigaSure may be used to divide the mesentery up to the edge of the bowel. This may be done before freeing the lateral attachments of the sigmoid and left colon as it aids in retraction.

After division of the mesentery, the lateral attachments of the sigmoid to the abdominal wall are divided along the white line. Care is taken to avoid damage to the retroperitoneal structures.

The colon is then divided using a linear endoscopic stapler at the site where the colonic mesentery has been divided.

RECTAL MOBILIZATION

In women, the uterus may be hitched out of the area of dissection with a suture (see Figure 5E.4). Atraumatic bowel clamps that are inserted through the left-sided ports are used to elevate the rectosigmoid colon out of the pelvis and away from the retroperitoneum and sacral promontory, to enable entry into the presacral space. The posterior aspect of the mesorectum can be identified and the mesorectal plane dissected with diathermy, preserving the hypogastric nerves passing down into the pelvis anterior to the sacrum. Dissection continues down the presacral space in this avascular plane toward the pelvic floor. Attention is now switched to the peritoneum on the right side of the rectum (see Figure 5E.5). This is divided to the level of the seminal vesicles or rectovaginal septum. This is repeated on the peritoneum on the left side of the rectum (see Figure 5E.6). This facilitates further posterior dissection along the back of the mesorectum to the pelvic floor, to a level inferior to the lower edge of the mesorectum. Usually, when the approach is low on the posterior surface of the mesorectum, it becomes necessary to perform a lateral and anterior dissection (see Figure 5E.7).

A bowel grasper inserted through the left iliac fossa port is used to retract the peritoneum anterior to the rectum forward. The peritoneal dissection is continued from the free edge of the lateral peritoneal dissection, anteriorly. Lateral dissection is continued on both sides of the rectum and is extended anterior to the rectum in front of Denonvillier's fascia, separating the posterior vaginal wall from the anterior wall of the rectum or down past the level of the prostate in men (see Figures 5E.8–5E.10). The most inferior rectal dissection can be completed from the perineal approach. For anterior tumors, the dissection may be performed anterior to Denonvillier's fascia, or by taking one side of the fascia to protect the anterolateral nerve bundle.

It is necessary to perform a total mesorectal excision and hence the rectum must be dissected down close to the muscle tube of the rectum below the level of the mesorectum. The levators may then be divided from above, staying well wide of any potential tumor, or the division may be performed from below after making the perineal incision (see Figure 5E.11).

FORMATION OF TREPHINE LEFT ILIAC FOSSA COLOSTOMY

The divided distal end of the left sigmoid colon is grasped with atraumatic bowel clamps, which are locked. A trephine colostomy is made in the left iliac fossa at a site that has been marked by an enterostomal therapist before surgery. A skin disk is excised, and a longitudinal incision is made in the anterior rectus sheath and the left rectus muscle is split. The peritoneum is held with two hemostats and incised. The stapled colon is delivered to the trephine and grasped with Babcock forceps and delivered through the trephine. The staple line is excised and the end colostomy is matured using 3/0 chromic catgut sutures.

PERINEAL DISSECTION

The perineal dissection is performed with a conventional open approach. The anus is sutured closed with 0 nylon and an elliptical skin incision is made. The incision is deepened using diathermy and the ischiorectal fossae are entered on either side, well lateral to the external sphincter muscle. The dissection continues laterally and posteriorly to expose the levator ani muscles. The tip of the coccyx is used as the posterior landmark and the pelvic cavity is entered by dividing the levator ani muscle just anterior to the tip of the coccyx. A finger can be placed into the pelvis onto the upper border of levator ani, which is divided with diathermy onto the underlying finger. Care is taken anteriorly to divide the remaining levator ani while protecting the posterior surface of the vagina or prostate/urethra. The specimen may then be delivered out of the pelvis, which facilitates division of the remaining anterior attachments of the rectum, reducing the risk of damage to the prostate or posterior wall of the vagina. The specimen is removed, the pelvic cavity irrigated of blood or debris, and the perineal tissue closed in layers using polydioxanone sutures.

PORT SITE CLOSURE

The right iliac fossa 12-mm port site is closed using an ENDO CLOSE (see Chapter 4I). The umbilical port site is closed using the previously inserted purse-string suture.

F | HARTMANN REVERSAL 💿

KEY STEPS

1. Peristomal incision for stoma mobilization; 0 polypropylene purse-string suture and insertion of circular stapler anvil into distal end of colon.

2. Insertion of ports: 12-mm open technique through stoma site after mobilization of stoma; 10-mm at umbilicus for camera; 5-mm right iliac fossa; 5-mm right upper quadrant; 5-mm left upper quadrant if necessary.

3. Patient in Trendelenburg (slight rotation to right may be required to aid visualization of sacral promontory).

4. Laparoscopic assessment, and small bowel and omentum moved toward right upper quadrant. Adhesiolysis as needed to identify rectal stump.

5. Lateral mobilization of left colon and splenic flexure to allow tension-free reach of colon to rectum. Left ureter identified.

6. Medial-to-lateral mobilization of sigmoid colon off Gerota's fascia.

7. Rectal mobilization (only necessary if distal sigmoid still present or stapler cannot be advanced transanally). Dissection in the presacral plane to free proximal rectum with preservation of hypogastric nerves (no violation of fascia propria of rectum).

8. Circular stapled anastomosis completed and leak test performed.

9. Closure of all trocar sites >5 mm.

PATIENT POSITIONING

The patient is placed supine on the operating table, on a beanbag. After induction of general anesthesia and insertion of an orogastric tube and Foley catheter, the legs are placed in Dan Allen or Yellowfin stirrups (see Figure 5F.1). The arms are tucked at the patient's side and the beanbag is aspirated. The abdomen is prepared with antiseptic solution and draped routinely (see Chapter 4).

INSTRUMENT POSITIONING

The primary monitor is placed on the left side of the patient at approximately the level of the hip. The secondary monitor is placed on the right side of the patient at the same level, and is primarily for the assistant during the early phase of the surgery and port insertion (see Figure 5F.2). The operating nurse's instrument table is placed between the patient's legs. There should be sufficient space to allow the surgeon to move from either

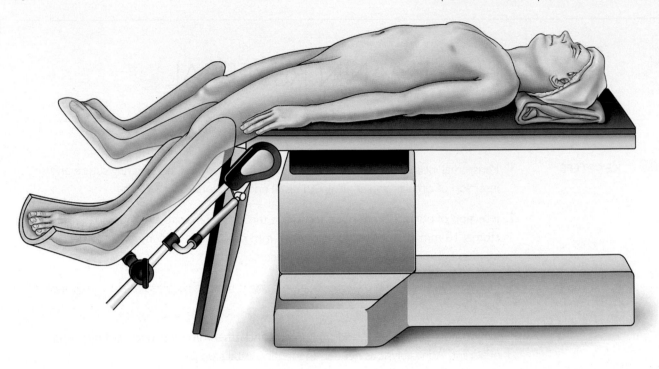

Figure 5F.1 The patient is positioned on the table in Dan Allen stirrups.

side of the patient to between the patient's legs, if necessary. The primary operating surgeon stands on the right side of the patient with the assistant standing on the patient's left, and moving to the right side, caudad to the surgeon once ports have been inserted. A 0-degree camera lens is used.

LAPAROSCOPY AND INSERTION OF REMAINING PORTS

The colostomy is mobilized and all adhesions dissected through the fascial opening until an adequate segment of bowel has been freed from the surrounding tissues. The bowel is trimmed as necessary and a purse-string suture is positioned before insertion of the anvil of a curved EEA stapling device. The bowel is returned to the abdomen, the fascia is closed with a monofilament suture, but before tying the suture a 12-mm port is inserted at this site, and the abdomen is insufflated.

The camera is inserted into the abdomen through the stoma trocar to assess adhesions and allow direct visualization for subsequent trocar insertion and an initial laparoscopy is performed, carefully evaluating the liver, small bowel, and peritoneal surfaces. A 10-mm port is inserted in the umbilicus for camera location. A 5-mm right lower quadrant trocar is placed approximately 2 to 3 cm medial to the anterior superior iliac spine. This is carefully inserted lateral to the inferior epigastric vessels, paying attention to keep the tract of the port going as perpendicular as possible through the abdominal wall. A 5-mm port is then inserted in the right upper quadrant at least a hand's breadth superior to the lower quadrant port. A left upper quadrant 5-mm port is

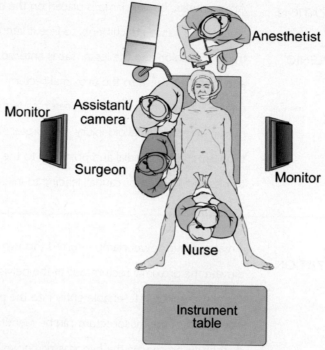

Figure 5F.2 Operating room setup for sigmoid procedures.

inserted. Again all of these remaining ports are kept lateral to the epigastric vessels. This may be ensured by diligence to anatomic port site selection and using the laparoscope to transilluminate the abdominal wall before making the port site incision to identify any obvious superficial vessels.

DEFINITIVE LAPARO-SCOPIC SETUP

The assistant now moves to the patient's right side, standing caudad to the surgeon. The patient is rotated with the left side up and right side down, to approximately 15 to 20 degrees tilt, and often as far as the table can go. This helps to move the small bowel over to the right side of the abdomen. The patient is then placed in the Trendelenburg position. This again helps gravitational migration of the small bowel away from the operative field. The surgeon then inserts two atraumatic bowel clamps through the two right-sided abdominal ports. The greater omentum is reflected over the transverse colon so that it comes to lie on the stomach. If there is no space in the upper part of the abdomen, one must confirm that the orogastric tube is adequately decompressing the stomach. The small bowel is moved to the patient's right side allowing visualization of the proximal rectum. Variable degrees of adhesiolysis may be required. This may necessitate the use of the assistant's 5-mm atraumatic bowel clamp through the stoma trocar or left upper quadrant.

MOBILIZATION OF LEFT COLON AND SPLENIC FLEXURE

An atraumatic bowel clamp is placed on the descending colon to take down the inflammatory and native attachments to free it laterally. The omentum is dissected off the transverse colon and the lesser sac is entered. The splenic flexure is released to allow a tension-free reach to the proximal rectum. The colonic mesentery should be mobilized off the Gerota's fascia. The left ureter is identified at the pelvic brim and freed from the proximal rectum to avoid injury. The ureter should be just deep to the parietal peritoneum, and just medial and posterior to the gonadal vessels. Care must be taken not to dissect too deep or caudal, leading to injury of the iliac vessels.

RECTAL MOBILIZATION

An atraumatic bowel clamp inserted through the left lower quadrant port is used to elevate the proximal rectum out of the pelvis and away from the retroperitoneum and sacral promontory, to enable entry into the presacral space (see Figure 5F.3). The posterior aspect of the mesorectum can be identified and the mesorectal plane dissected with diathermy, preserving the hypogastric nerves as they pass down into the pelvis anterior to the sacrum. Dissection needs to progress only to allow advancement of the circular stapler to the end of the rectum and assure that all the sigmoid has been resected. If residual sigmoid is present (see Figure 5F.4), the linear endoscopic stapler should be used to divide the bowel at the level of the proximal rectum. A site for rectal division should be chosen in proximal, peritonealized rectum, which assures that the anastomosis will be distal to the sacral promontory. The rectum is divided laparoscopically with a linear endoscopic stapler through the right lower quadrant trocar. One or two firings of the stapler may be required to divide the rectum. The mesorectum is divided using monopolar and bipolar cautery at this level.

SPECIMEN EXTRACTION AND ANASTOMOSIS

If residual sigmoid is required, the specimen is extracted through the stoma site trocar. Pneumoperitoneum is recreated, and the circular stapled anastomosis is formed under laparoscopic guidance (see Figures 5F.5–5F.7). The anastomosis can be leak-tested by filling the pelvis with saline and inflating the neorectum using a proctoscope or bulb syringe and the orientation and lack of tension confirmed (see Figure 5F.8).

PORT SITE CLOSURE

Port site closure techniques are discussed in Chapter 4I. The umbilical port site is closed using the previously inserted purse-string suture.

G | RESECTION RECTOPEXY 📀

KEY STEPS

1. Insertion of ports: 10-mm umbilical open technique; 12-mm right iliac fossa; 5-mm right upper quadrant; 5-mm left iliac fossa.

2. Patient in Trendelenburg (slight rotation to right may be required to aid visualization of sacral promontory).

3. Laparoscopic assessment, and small bowel and omentum moved towards right upper quadrant.

4. Inferior mesenteric artery pedicle identified from medial aspect and elevated off retroperitoneum. Left ureter identified and inferior mesenteric artery divided distal to take of left colic artery.

5. Medial-to-lateral mobilization of sigmoid colon with little dissection of descending colon.

6. Lateral paracolic mobilization of sigmoid colon but limited mobilization of left colon.

7. Rectal mobilization. Dissection behind the posterior 60% of the rectum in the presacral plane (no violation of fascia propria of rectum).

8. Division of peritoneal attachments on right and left side of rectum to the level of the lateral stalks (should be preserved).

9. No anterior dissection of rectum, unless required to completely reduce a distal prolapse.

10. Rectum stapled proximally in the peritonealized segment at a level that assures anastomosis rostral to sacral promontory.

11. Extracorporeal resection of descending colon–sigmoid colon junction through muscle-splitting incision at left lower quadrant trocar site.

12. Closure of left lower quadrant wound and intracorporeal circular stapled colorectal anastomosis under laparoscopic guidance.

13. Elevation of rectum out of pelvis under appropriate tension and suture rectopexy of the right side of the mesorectum (distal to the anastomosis) to sacral promontory using permanent suture.

14. Closure of ports >5 mm in size.

PATIENT POSITIONING

The patient is placed supine on the operating table, on a beanbag. After induction of general anesthesia and insertion of an oro-gastric tube and Foley catheter, the legs are placed in Dan Allen or Yellowfin stirrups (see Figure 5G.1). The arms are tucked at the

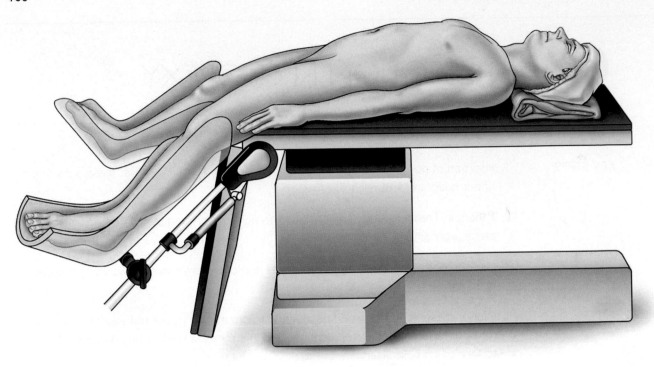

Figure 5G.1 The patient is positioned on the table in Dan Allen stirrups.

patient's side and the beanbag is aspirated. The abdomen is prepared with antiseptic solution and draped routinely (see Chapter 4).

INSTRUMENT POSITIONING

The primary monitor is placed on the left side of the patient at approximately the level of the hip. The secondary monitor is placed on the right side of the patient at the same level, and is primarily for the assistant during the early phase of the surgery and port insertion (see Figure 5G.2). The operating nurse's instrument table is placed between the patient's legs. There should be sufficient space to allow the surgeon to move from either side of the patient to between the patient's legs, if necessary. The primary operating surgeon stands on the right side of the patient with the assistant standing on the patient's left, and moving to the right side, caudad to the surgeon once ports have been inserted. A 0-degree camera lens is used.

UMBILICAL PORT INSERTION

This is performed using a modified Hasson approach (see Chapter 4). A vertical 1-cm subumbilical incision is made. This is deepened down to the linea alba, which is then grasped on each side of the midline using Kocher clamps. A scalpel (No. 15 blade) is used to open the fascia between the Kocher clamps and a Kelly forceps is used to open the peritoneum bluntly. It is important to keep this opening small (<1 cm) to minimize air leaks. Having confirmed entry into the peritoneal cavity, a purse-string suture of

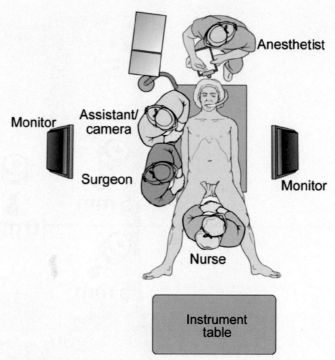

Figure 5G.2 Operating room setup for sigmoid procedures.

0 polyglycolic acid is placed around the subumbilical fascial defect (umbilical port site) and a Rommel tourniquet is applied. A 10-mm reusable port is inserted through this port site allowing the abdomen to be insufflated with CO_2 to a pressure of 12 mm Hg.

LAPAROSCOPY AND INSERTION OF REMAINING PORTS

The camera is inserted into the abdomen and an initial laparoscopy is performed, carefully evaluating the liver, small bowel, and peritoneal surfaces. A 12-mm port is inserted in the right lower quadrant approximately 2 to 3 cm medial and superior to the anterior superior iliac spine (see Figure 5G.3). This is carefully inserted lateral to the inferior epigastric vessels, paying attention to keep the tract of the port going as perpendicular as possible through the abdominal wall. A 5-mm port is then inserted in the right upper quadrant at least a hand's breadth superior to the lower quadrant port. A left lower quadrant 5-mm port is inserted. Again, all of these remaining ports are kept lateral to the epigastric vessels. This may be ensured by diligence to anatomical port site selection and using the laparoscope to transilluminate the abdominal wall before making the port site incision to identify any obvious superficial vessels.

DEFINITIVE LAPARO-SCOPIC SETUP

The assistant now moves to the patient's left side, standing caudad to the surgeon. The patient is rotated with the left side up and right side down, to approximately 15 to 20 degrees tilt, and often as far as the table can go. This helps to move the small bowel over to the right side of the abdomen. The patient is then placed in the Trendelenburg position.

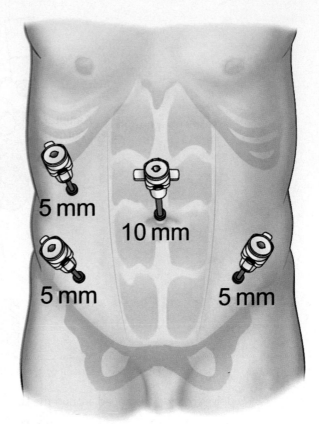

Figure 5G.3 Port setup for rectopexy.

This again helps gravitational migration of the small bowel away from the operative field. The surgeon then inserts two atraumatic bowel clamps through the two right-sided abdominal ports. The greater omentum is reflected over the transverse colon so that it comes to lie on the stomach. If there is no space in the upper part of the abdomen one must confirm that the orogastric tube is adequately decompressing the stomach. The small bowel is moved to the patient's right side allowing visualization of the medial aspect of the rectosigmoid mesentery. This may necessitate the use of the assistant's 5-mm atraumatic bowel clamp through the left lower quadrant to tent the sigmoid mesentery cephalad.

DEFINING AND DIVIDING THE INFERIOR MESENTERIC PEDICLE

An atraumatic bowel clamp is placed on the rectosigmoid mesentery at the level of the sacral promontory, approximately half way between the bowel wall and the promontory itself. This area is then stretched up towards the left lower quadrant port, stretching the inferior mesenteric vessels away from the retroperitoneum. In most cases, this demonstrates a groove between the right or medial side of the inferior mesenteric pedicle and the retroperitoneum. Cautery is used to open the peritoneum along this line, opening the plane cranially up to the origin of the inferior mesenteric artery, and caudally past the sacral promontory. Blunt dissection is then used to lift the vessels away from the retroperitoneum and presacral autonomic nerves. The ureter is then looked for under the inferior mesenteric artery. If the ureter cannot be seen, and the dissection is in the correct plane, the ureter should be just deep to the parietal peritoneum, and just medial to the gonadal vessels. Care must be taken not to dissect too deep or caudal leading to injury of the iliac vessels.

If the ureter cannot be found, it has usually been elevated on the back of the inferior mesenteric pedicle, and one needs to stay very close to the vessel not only to find the ureter but also to protect the autonomic nerves. If the ureter still cannot be found, the dissection needs to come in a cranial dissection, which is usually into clean tissue allowing it to be found. If this fails, a lateral approach can be performed (see subsequent text). This usually gives a fresh perspective to the tissues, and the ureter can often be found quite easily. In very rare cases the ureter still may not be found. We do not use ureteric stents as a routine, so the options at this stage include conversion to open surgery, or insertion of ureteric stents. We do not proceed if the ureter cannot be defined. The dissection should allow sufficient mobilization of the inferior mesenteric artery so that the origin of the left colic artery is seen. The vessel is carefully defined and divided just distal to the left colic artery. A clamp is placed on the origin of the vessel to control it if clips or other energy sources do not adequately control the vessel. In general, a cartridge of the endoscopic linear stapler is used to divide the vessel. This helps minimize expenditure, as the stapler will anyway be required for division of the rectum. Laparoscopic clips or other energy sources may also be used.

Having divided the pedicle, the plane between the sigmoid colon mesentery and the retroperitoneum is developed laterally, out towards the lateral attachment of the colon. Limited mobilization of the mesentery off the anterior surface of Gerota's fascia and of the left colon should be performed to enhance fixation of the rectum.

MOBILIZATION OF THE LATERAL ATTACHMENTS OF THE RECTOSIGMOID

The surgeon now grasps the rectosigmoid junction with his left-hand instrument and draws it to the patient's right side. This allows the lateral attachments of the sigmoid colon to be seen and divided using cautery. Bruising from the prior retroperitoneal mobilization of the colon can usually be seen in this area. Once this layer of peritoneum has been opened, one immediately enters into the space opened by the retroperitoneal dissection. No dissection should be performed more proximally along the white line of Toldt, toward the splenic flexure.

RECTAL MOBILIZATION

An atraumatic bowel clamp inserted through the left lower quadrant port is used to elevate the rectosigmoid colon out of the pelvis and away from the retroperitoneum and sacral promontory, to enable entry into the presacral space. The posterior aspect of the mesorectum can be identified and the mesorectal plane dissected with diathermy, preserving the hypogastric nerves as they pass down into the pelvis anterior to the sacrum. Dissection continues down the presacral space in this avascular plane toward the pelvic floor. Only the posterior 60% of the rectum needs to be mobilized; however, dissection should be continued all the way to the levator ani muscles. A transanal examining finger should be used to confirm the distal extent of the dissection. The lateral stalks should be preserved. The peritoneum on either side of the rectum should be incised to the level of the lateral stalks. The lateral stalks should generally be preserved, the exception being when further dissection must completely reduce a very distal prolapsing segment.

RECTAL DIVISION

The fully mobilized rectum should be elevated out of the pelvis and a site selected for optimal rectal tension to maintain full reduction of the prolapse. A site for rectal division should be chosen in proximal, peritonealized rectum, which assures that the anastomosis will be rostral to the sacral promontory. The rectum is divided laparoscopically with a linear endoscopic stapler through the right lower quadrant trocar. One or two firings of the stapler may be required to divide the rectum. The mesorectum is divided using monopolar and bipolar cautery at this level.

SPECIMEN EXTRACTION AND ANASTOMOSIS

The specimen is extracted through a left iliac fossa incision. Before making the incision, the proximal colonic transection point should be grasped with a locking atraumatic bowel grasper. This site should allow a colorectal anastomosis that will provide a safe amount of tension on the rectum to maintain prolapse reduction. After extracorporeal bowel transection, adequate vascularity of the colon should be assured.

A 2/0 Prolene purse-string suture is inserted into the distal end of the left colon, the anvil of a circular stapling gun is inserted, and the purse-string suture is tied tightly. The colon is returned to the abdomen and the left iliac fossa incision is closed in layers with 0 polyglycolic acid suture. Pneumoperitoneum is recreated, and the circular stapled anastomosis is formed under laparoscopic guidance. The anastomosis can be leak-tested by filling the pelvis with saline and inflating the neorectum using a proctoscope or bulb syringe.

RECTOPEXY

The rectum is retracted rostrally to the desired tension to allow complete reduction of the prolapse. The rectopexy is then performed from the right side using the two remaining trocars. Two or three nonabsorbable sutures are used to attach the mesorectum distal to the anastomosis to the sacral promontory. Alternatively, metal tacks may be employed using one of the mechanical fixation devices used for mesh hernia repairs.

PORT SITE CLOSURE

The right iliac fossa 12-mm port site is closed using an ENDO CLOSE (see Chapter 4I). The umbilical port site is closed using the previously inserted purse-string suture.

H | WELLS RECTOPEXY

KEY STEPS

1. Insertion of ports: 10-mm umbilical open technique; 5-mm right iliac fossa; 5-mm right upper quadrant; 5-mm left iliac fossa.

2. Patient in Trendelenburg (slight rotation to right may be required to aid visualization of sacral promontory).

3. Laparoscopic assessment, and small bowel and omentum moved toward right upper quadrant.

4. Inferior mesenteric artery pedicle identified from medial aspect and elevated off retroperitoneum. Left ureter is identified. No vascular division is performed.

5. Medial-to-lateral mobilization of sigmoid colon with little dissection of descending colon.

6. Lateral paracolic mobilization of sigmoid colon but limited mobilization of left colon.

7. Rectal mobilization. Dissection behind the posterior 60% of the rectum in the presacral plane (no violation of fascia propria of rectum).

8. Division of peritoneal attachments on right and left side of rectum to the level of the lateral stalks (should be preserved).

9. No anterior dissection of rectum.

10. Insertion of a 2 × 4 cm piece of polypropylene mesh through the umbilical trocar and positioned at the sacral promontory. Fixation of the mesh to the promontory.

11. Elevation of rectum out of pelvis under appropriate tension and suture rectopexy of the mesorectum to the mesh.

12. Closure of umbilical port fascia.

PATIENT POSITIONING

The patient is placed supine on the operating table, on a beanbag. After induction of general anesthesia and insertion of an oral gastric tube and Foley catheter, the legs are placed in Dan Allen or Yellow fin stirrups (see Figure 5H.1). The arms are tucked at the

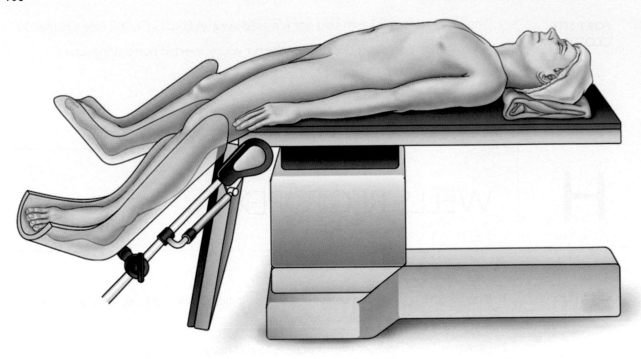

Figure 5H.1 The patient is positioned on the table in Dan Allen stirrups.

patient's side and the beanbag is aspirated. The abdomen is prepared with antiseptic solution and draped routinely (see Chapter 4).

INSTRUMENT POSITIONING

The primary monitor is placed on the left side of the patient at approximately the level of the hip. The secondary monitor is placed on the right side of the patient at the same level, and is primarily for the assistant during the early phase of the surgery and port insertion (see Figure 5H.2). The operating nurse's instrument table is placed between the patient's legs. There should be sufficient space to allow the surgeon to move from either side of the patient to between the patient's legs, if necessary. The primary operating surgeon stands on the right side of the patient with the assistant standing on the patient's left, and moving to the right side, caudad to the surgeon once ports have been inserted. A 0-degree camera lens is used.

UMBILICAL PORT INSERTION

This is performed using a modified Hasson approach (see Chapter 4). A vertical 1-cm subumbilical incision is made. This is deepened down to the linea alba, which is then grasped on each side of the midline using Kocher clamps. A scalpel (No. 15 blade) is used to open the fascia between the Kocher clamps and a Kelly forceps is used to open the peritoneum bluntly. It is important to keep this opening small (<1 cm) to minimize air leaks. Having confirmed entry into the peritoneal cavity, a purse-string suture of 0 polyglycolic acid is placed around the subumbilical fascial defect (umbilical port site)

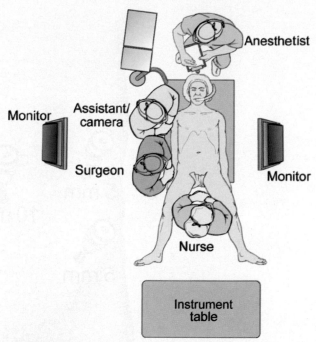

Figure 5H.2 Operating room setup for sigmoid procedures.

and a Rommel tourniquet is applied. A 10-mm reusable port is inserted through this port site allowing the abdomen to be insufflated with CO_2 to a pressure of 12 mm Hg.

LAPAROSCOPY AND INSERTION OF REMAINING PORTS

The camera is inserted into the abdomen and an initial laparoscopy is performed, carefully evaluating the liver, small bowel, and peritoneal surfaces. A 5-mm port is inserted in the right lower quadrant approximately 2 to 3 cm medial and superior to the anterior superior iliac spine (see Figure 5H.3). This is carefully inserted lateral to the inferior epigastric vessels, paying attention to keep the tract of the port going as perpendicular as possible through the abdominal wall. A 5-mm port is then inserted in the right upper quadrant at least a hand's breadth superior to the lower quadrant port. A left lower quadrant 5-mm port is inserted. Again, all of these remaining ports are kept lateral to the epigastric vessels. This may be ensured by diligence to anatomic port site selection and using the laparoscope to transilluminate the abdominal wall before making the port site incision to identify any obvious superficial vessels.

DEFINITIVE LAPARO-SCOPIC SETUP

The assistant now moves to the patient's left side, standing caudad to the surgeon. The patient is rotated with the left side up and right side down, to approximately 15 to 20 degrees tilt, and often as far as the table can go. This helps to move the small bowel over to the right side of the abdomen. The patient is then placed in the Trendelenburg position. This again helps gravitational migration of the small bowel away from the operative field. The

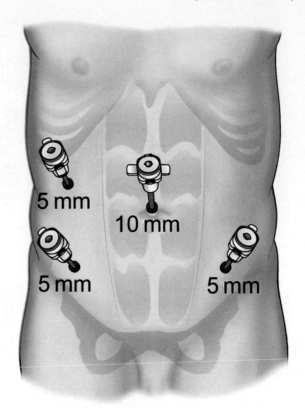

Figure 5H.3 Port setup for rectopexy.

surgeon then inserts two atraumatic bowel clamps through the two right-sided abdominal ports. The greater omentum is reflected over the transverse colon so that it comes to lie on the stomach. If there is no space in the upper part of the abdomen, one must confirm that the orogastric tube is adequately decompressing the stomach. The small bowel is moved to the patient's right side allowing visualization of the medial aspect of the rectosigmoid mesentery. This may necessitate the use of the assistant's 5-mm atraumatic bowel clamp through the left lower quadrant to tent the sigmoid mesentery cephalad.

DEFINING THE INFERIOR MESENTERIC PEDICLE

An atraumatic bowel clamp is placed on the rectosigmoid mesentery at the level of the sacral promontory, approximately half way between the bowel wall and the promontory itself. This area is then stretched up toward the left lower quadrant port, stretching the inferior mesenteric vessels away from the retroperitoneum. In most cases, this demonstrates a groove between the right or medial side of the inferior mesenteric pedicle and the retroperitoneum. Cautery is used to open the peritoneum along this line, opening the plane cranially up to the origin of the inferior mesenteric artery, and caudally past the sacral promontory (see Figure 5H.4). Blunt dissection is then used to lift the vessels away from the retroperitoneum and presacral autonomic nerves (see Figure 5H.5). The ureter is then looked for under the inferior mesenteric artery. If the ureter cannot be seen, and the dissection is in the correct plane, the ureter should be just deep to the parietal peritoneum, and just medial to the gonadal vessels. Care must be taken not to dissect too deep or caudal, leading to injury of the iliac vessels.

If the ureter cannot be found, it has usually been elevated on the back of the inferior mesenteric pedicle, and one needs to stay very close to the vessel not only to find the ureter but also to protect the autonomic nerves. If the ureter still cannot be found, the dissection needs to come in a cranial dissection, which is usually into clean tissue allowing it to be found. If this fails, a lateral approach can be performed (see subsequent text). This usually gives a fresh perspective to the tissues, and the ureter can often be found quite easily. In very rare cases, the ureter still may not be found. We do not use ureteric stents as a routine, so the options at this stage include conversion to open surgery, or insertion of ureteric stents. We do not proceed if the ureter cannot be defined. The dissection should allow sufficient mobilization of the inferior mesenteric artery so that the origin of the left colic artery is seen. The pedicle is not divided.

The plane between the sigmoid colon mesentery and the retroperitoneum is developed laterally, out toward the lateral attachment of the colon. Limited mobilization of the mesentery off the anterior surface of Gerota's fascia and of the left colon should be performed to enhance fixation of the rectum.

MOBILIZATION OF THE LATERAL ATTACHMENTS OF THE RECTOSIGMOID

The surgeon now grasps the rectosigmoid junction with his left-hand instrument and draws it to the patient's right side. This allows the lateral attachments of the sigmoid colon to be seen and divided using cautery. Bruising from the prior retroperitoneal mobilization of the colon can usually be seen in this area. Once this layer of peritoneum has been opened, one immediately enters into the space opened by the retroperitoneal dissection. No dissection should be performed more proximally along the white line of Toldt, toward the splenic flexure.

RECTAL MOBILIZATION

An atraumatic bowel clamp inserted through the left lower quadrant port is used to elevate the rectosigmoid colon out of the pelvis and away from the retroperitoneum and sacral promontory, to enable entry into the presacral space. The posterior aspect of the mesorectum can be identified and the mesorectal plane dissected with diathermy, preserving the hypogastric nerves as they pass down into the pelvis anterior to the sacrum. Dissection continues down the presacral space in this avascular plane toward the pelvic floor (see Figure 5H.6). Only the posterior 60% of the rectum needs be mobilized; however, dissection should be continued all the way to the levator ani muscles. A transanal examining finger should be used to confirm the distal extent of the dissection.

The peritoneum on either side of the rectum should be incised to the level of the lateral stalks (see Figure 5H.7). The lateral stalks should generally be preserved, the exception being when further dissection must completely reduce a very distal prolapsing segment (see Figure 5H.8). The rectum is not divided.

RECTOPEXY

A 2 × 4 cm portion of polypropylene mesh is rolled and inserted through the umbilical trocar. The camera is reinserted and the mesh is positioned at the sacral promontory (see Figure 5H.9). A mechanical device used for hernia mesh fixation is used to fix the mesh to the promontory. This may be inserted through the right lower quadrant port, but if adequate access cannot be obtained, a 5-mm suprapubic port may be inserted. Great care must be taken not to tear or strip off the presacral fascia when stapling the mesh in place.

The rectum is retracted rostrally to the desired tension to allow complete reduction of the prolapse, which is confirmed by digital rectal examination. The rectopexy is then performed from the right side using the two right-sided trocars. Two or three nonabsorbable sutures are used to attach the distal mesorectum to the mesh at the promontory, sufficient to maintain adequate tension. Alternatively, the mechanical fixation device used for mesh fixation may be employed. If the left side of the mesorectum is also being fixed to the mesh, this is performed before doing the right side, as access is easier when the left is performed first (see Figures 5H.10–5H.12).

PORT SITE CLOSURE

The umbilical port site is closed using the previously inserted purse-string suture. The remaining 5-mm ports are removed.

TOTAL COLECTOMY

I | SUBTOTAL COLECTOMY AND ILEORECTAL ANASTOMOSIS

KEY STEPS

1. Patient positioning.

2. Insertion of ports: 10-mm umbilical Hasson technique; 12-mm right iliac fossa; 5-mm right upper quadrant; 5-mm left upper quadrant; 5 to 10 mm left iliac fossa.

3. Instrument positioning and laparoscopic assessment.

4. Laparoscopic mobilization of right colon and terminal ileum.

5. Laparoscopic mobilization of transverse colon and take down of splenic flexure.

6. Division of middle colic vessels.

7. Laparoscopic mobilization of left colon.

8. Mobilization and division of upper rectum, mesorectum, and descending colonic mesentery.

9. Confirmation of colonic mobility.

10. Exteriorization of specimen and preservation of mesenteric orientation.

11. Reinsufflation and anastomosis.

12. Port closure.

PATIENT POSITIONING

The correct positioning of the patient is of utmost importance when undertaking any laparoscopic resections but this is particularly true when mobilization of the transverse colon is necessitated. The patient undergoes general anaesthesia, with a Foley catheter and oral gastric tube in place. The patient is placed on a beanbag with both arms tucked at the sides. The lower aspect of the beanbag should not encroach over the "break" in the operating table and the patient's buttocks should rest on this edge permitting easy access for a standard circular stapler to be used transanally to complete the ileorectal anastomosis. The patient's legs are placed in stirrups and in compression pneumatic stockings (see Figure 51.1). The popliteal angle is maintained with slight flexion of the knee joint and the hip joint is supine with a slight extension and abduction if possible. The correct positioning of the lower limbs is essential as access to the transverse colon is significantly impeded if the quadriceps is bulky or if there is any hip flexion.

PORT INSERTION

There are five port sites used for a subtotal colectomy (see Figure 51.2). The initial port site is an infraumbilical 10-mm port. This is the camera port and a good pneumatic seal is essential at this port site. A modified Hasson technique is used and described in detail in Chapter 4. Briefly, a 1-cm infraumbilical vertical incision is made with a No. 11 blade and the incision is deepened to expose the linea alba. The linea is grasped between two Kocher forceps and an incision is made with a Mayo scissors to breach the linea and underlying peritoneum. The entry into the peritoneal cavity is confirmed with a blunt

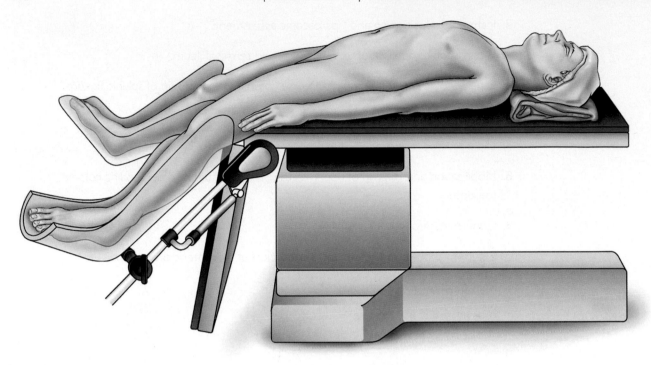

Figure 51.1 The patient is positioned on the table in Dan Allen stirrups.

artery forceps (Kelly forceps), which should slide easily into the peritoneal cavity. A 0 polyglycolic acid purse-string suture is then used to secure the linea and aid in maintaining an effective seal. The 10-mm port is inserted and the pneumoperitoneum is established. The remaining ports are located in the right and left upper quadrants and these are both 5-mm port sites. These are positioned a comfortable hand's breadth superiorly from their corresponding lower ports (12–15 cm). The positioning of these upper quadrant ports should avoid impedance of the lower costal margin and avoid potential "fencing" with their ipsilateral lower port. The lower port sites are located "1 inch in and 1 inch up" (medially and cephalad) from the corresponding anterior superior iliac spine. A 12-mm port site is used for the right lower quadrant to permit an endoscopic gastrointestinal stapler to be inserted for division of the rectum. A 5-mm left lower quadrant port is used to permit use of a harmonic ultrasonic instrument or a LigaSure bipolar instrument when ligating the ileocolic pedicle and middle colic vessels, as this has been our practice due to the number of vessels being divided. This port site may necessarily be 10 mm in size if one uses a 10-mm harmonic scalpel or the LigaSure device.

INSTRUMENT POSITIONING AND LAPARO-SCOPIC ASSESSMENT

The case is dependent on having two monitors (see Figures 51.3 and 51.4). They are initially located on each side of the upper quadrants. The patient is prepped and draped to permit lateral access to the port sites. There should be two instrument-holding "quivers." These are attached one on each side to the lateral aspect of the

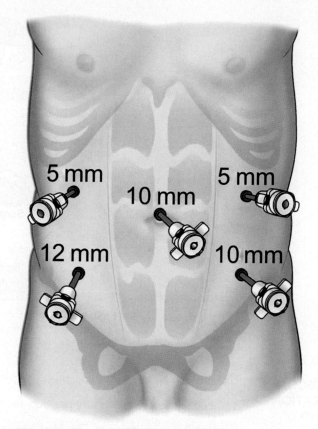

Figure 51.2 Port setup for total colectomy.

patient's thighs. They contain two bowel-grasping forceps in each quiver and the dissecting electrocautery scissors, irrigation suction device, harmonic scalpel, or LigaSure instruments. The operating nurse should set up the instrument table opposite the patient's feet and allow sufficient space for the surgeon to move from right or left to between the legs as the case progresses. A 0-degree camera lens is used; however, a 30-degree lens or a flexible tip lens may be used with equal efficacy and may be particularly useful if there is a high splenic flexure or other anatomic variant. The initial assessment is a complete laparoscopy of the abdominal contents. Minor median adhesions obstructing assessment of the abdominal cavity should be dissected free and any unexpected pathology noted. The sequence of the procedure begins with the mobilization of the right colon and the terminal ileum in its entirety. The surgeon stands on the patient's left side at the level of the patient's hips. The surgical assistant stands on the surgeon's right side toward the patient's head and holds the camera. A second assistant is used in these cases and he/she in turn stands opposite to the primary operating surgeon on the patient's right side, although the second assistant is generally needed only during mobilization of the transverse colon.

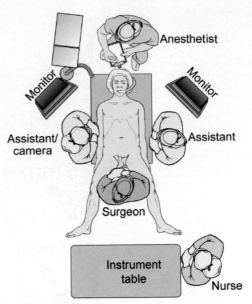

Figure 51.3 Operating room setup for total colectomy with the surgeon positioned between the patient's legs.

LAPAROSCOPIC MOBILIZATION OF RIGHT COLON AND TERMINAL ILEUM

The surgeon initially uses two bowel graspers to expose the ileocolic pedicle. The patient is placed in the Trendelenburg position and the greater omentum is reflected cephalad over the liver and stomach. The small bowel migrates to the upper abdomen with the patient turning to the Trendelenburg position and the remaining loops are placed in the left upper quadrant and left side of the abdomen. This facilitates exposure of the terminal ileum and this final aspect of the small bowel is best moved to the left lower quadrant to expose the mesentery of the ileocolic pedicle. In the event of difficulty,

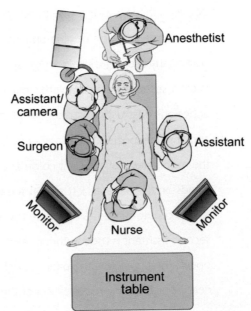

Figure 51.4 Operating room setup for total colectomy with the surgeon positioned on the right side.

the patient may also be tilted toward the surgeon to allow ileal loops to fall to the left side away from the initial operating field. The assistant standing opposite to the surgeon using a 5-mm bowel grasper secures the ileocecal junction and elevates this laterally and toward the right lower quadrant. This has the effect of the ileocolic vascular pedicle been drawn up from the retroperitoneum demonstrating the line of the vessels. The surgeon holds a bowel grasper in his left hand and electrocautery in his right hand and incises along the line of the exposed vessels. The bowel grasper is used to help correctly identify the potential fusion line between the retroperitoneum and underside of the ascending colonic mesentery. This is an avascular plane. Once the peritoneum has been opened, there is little need for any further sharp dissection to create this virtual space. This blunt dissection continues using traction and countertraction opening up the underside of the ascending colonic mesentery laterally and exposing the second part of the duodenum medially. The optimal movement is generally to elevate the ascending colon mesentery with the left-hand instrument and dissect or separate tissues off this plane with the right-hand instrument (see Figure 51.5).

The ileocolic pedicle should be exposed and a potential avascular window appears between the superior/lateral aspect of the base of the ileocolic pedicle and the duodenum. The surgeon now uses the bowel grasper to elevate this avascular window from the superior aspect (superficial) and using sharp dissection incises through into the virtual space opened up on the underside of the ascending colonic mesentery. The surgeon now places his scissors under the ileocolic pedicle and out through this newly created window and confirms its suitability for ligation. The ileocolic pedicle is then divided. This technique is outlined in detail in Chapter 4D. The assistant now drops the ileocecal junction and grasps the distal end of the transected ileocolic pedicle. The assistant elevates this along with the mesentery and the surgeon progressively bluntly dissects under the ascending mesentery to reach the lateral abdominal wall, the lower aspect of the liver, and the underside of the transverse colonic mesentery. It is important to dissect as far medially under the transverse colon while avoiding any duodenal or pancreatic injury. A low-rising right colic artery, or right branch of middle colic may be encountered while dissecting cephalad and this should be ligated with surgical clips, harmonic scalpel, or the LigaSure. The patient is now turned to reverse Trendelenburg and the surgeon enters into the peritoneal reflection between the proximal transverse colon and the lower border of the liver (see Figure 51.6). The assistant holds the colon just proximal to the hepatic flexure and draws it inferiorly toward the right lower quadrant in the line of the ascending colon. The surgeon holds the proximal aspect of the transverse colon with a bowel grasper and draws it toward the left lower quadrant. This has the effect of tenting the peritoneal reflection above the colon and allows the surgeon to dissect through the tented peritoneum into the previously opened virtual space underneath. Care must be taken to avoid the duodenum, which lies directly under this point of dissection. The dissection is then carried from medial to lateral to mobilize the hepatic flexure using the superior approach. Once the hepatic flexure has been reached, the assistant draws the colon toward the left lower quadrant and the surgeon continues the dissection as far caudal as possible. This usually is as far as the pelvic brim. The patient is now returned to the Trendelenburg position and the surgeon dissects the terminal ileum free from its attachment on the pelvic brim. This is achieved by reflecting the small bowel cephalad and exposing the inferior aspect of the terminal ileum. The assistant grasps the appendix base and elevates the cecum medially and superiorly. The surgeon uses the scissors in the left hand and the graspers in the right to hold the terminal ileum superiorly and medially. The dissection is from the inferior aspect of the ileal mesentery and the terminal ileum is dissected free from the retroperitoneum. This connects the inferior aspect dissection and the previously performed superior colonic dissection. The colon is mobilized medially and the inferior ileal dissection is continued medially to expose the third part of the duodenum. The right ureter should be protected and should not be exposed if the retroperitoneum has not been breached. The surgeon needs to confirm that the right colon has been completely mobilized as far as the middle of the transverse colon. Any further peritoneal attachments of the proximal transverse colon are now easily divided and this completes the ascending colonic mobilization. Throughout the entire mobilization of the right colon, the surgeon uses the two left-sided ports and remains on the patient's left side.

LAPAROSCOPIC MOBILIZATION OF TRANSVERSE COLON AND TAKE DOWN OF SPLENIC FLEXURE

Mobilization of the transverse colon may be undertaken as a continuation of right colon mobilization, or may be undertaken after mobilizing the left colon. This is generally the most difficult and tedious part of a total colectomy. The patient is in the reverse Trendelenburg position. The surgeon stands between the patient's legs and holds a bowel grasper in the left hand and a harmonic scalpel or LigaSure in the right hand through the right and left lower quadrant ports. The camera assistant stands at the patient's right side and uses a bowel grasper through the right upper quadrant port. The second assistant stands at the patient's left side and uses a bowel grasper through the left upper quadrant port. For benign cases, the left side of the greater omentum is dissected off the colon, keeping the dissection in the avascular plane between the omentum and the bowel itself (see Figure 51.7). This leads to the splenic flexure and permits relatively easy mobilization in most cases.

The grasper in the right upper quadrant is used to elevate the omentum of the mid-transverse colon. The left upper quadrant port holds the gastrocolic omentum cephalad. This holds up the omentum like a curtain, and the surgeon essentially "releases" the bowel off the omentum using cautery or the energy source of choice. The surgeon uses the bowel grasper in the left hand and the scissors with cautery, or harmonic scalpel or LigaSure in the right hand. The transverse colon and gastrocolic omentum are drawn caudal and the lesser sac entered at the middle of the transverse colon, through the avascular plane. The omentum is dissected off the colon going out toward the splenic flexure (see Figure 51.8). The dissection usually continues just around the flexure to high descending colon. By rolling the patient to the right, the lateral attachments of the descending colon can be mobilized with cautery allowing the splenic flexure to be completely freed, as further demonstrated in Chapter 4G.

The surgeon now switches the instruments to continue dissection from the middle of the lesser sac to the right side. Depending on the individual anatomy, sometimes it is easier to remain in the avascular plane, and sometimes it is easier to perform progressive division and ligation of the gastrocolic omentum, until the hepatic flexure is reached. This is usually straightforward, as much of this mobilization has been already performed during the right colon mobilization. All attachments of the colon should now be divided, leaving the middle colic vessels as the last point of dissection.

DIVISION OF MIDDLE COLIC VESSELS

The transverse colon, similarly, is now quite mobile. In a manner very similar to that performed for elevation of the greater omentum, the upper quadrant ports are now used to elevate the transverse colon and tent it out toward the respective flexures. The surgeon holds the bowel grasper in the left hand and ligating instrument in the right. Initially, an opening is made in the transverse colon omentum to the lesser sac through the avascular window (see Figure 51.9). It is easy to be more posterior than expected and care must be taken not to damage the pancreas or fourth part of the duodenum.

The middle colic vessels are progressively ligated from the patient's left side to the right (see Figure 51.10). Each branch should be treated with care and proximal control of the vessel should be maintained at all times with the bowel grasper. Difficulty may arise from a larger greater omentum encroaching on the operative field and this should be reflected cephalad. It is essential that the vascular pedicle is confirmed before division as the superior mesenteric artery and vein lie deep to the dissection line and the pancreas is fully exposed as dissection progresses (see Figure 51.11).

LAPAROSCOPIC MOBILIZATION OF LEFT COLON

The surgeon now moves to the patient's right side with the camera assistant on the surgeon's left. The assistant stands opposite to the surgeon, on the patient's left side. The patient is placed in the Trendelenburg position and the small bowel is mobilized to the right upper quadrant. The base of the sigmoid mesentery is therefore exposed, similar to a sigmoid colectomy described in Chapter 5C. The patient may also be tilted slightly "left side up" toward the surgeon if further exposure is necessary. The surgeon uses the bowel grasper in the left hand and the scissors in the right. The assistant uses the bowel grasper through the left lower quadrant port site and holds the rectosigmoid mesentery, tented and cephalad. The surgeon incises along the line reflecting the inferior mesenteric artery from the retroperitoneum. The retroperitoneum is preserved and this avoids injury to the hypogastric nerves and sympathetic sacral plexus. The dissection is carried from medial to lateral under the inferior mesenteric artery and sigmoid mesentery. The surgeon should avoid progressing into the pelvis, as this is often an easy line of dissection to follow; however, aggressive mobilization of the rectum is not indicated in this surgery, unless a proctocolectomy is being performed. The key structures to identify are the left ureter and gonadal vessels. The sequence from medial to lateral is that of left ureter, left gonadal vessels, and psoas tendon. If the surgeon reaches the psoas tendon, then the ureter must be located more medially in the dissected field. The left ureter must be identified before further progress is being made and consideration of dividing any vessels. The surgeon progresses from medial to lateral in the dissection and this again is through traction and counter traction. There is no sharp dissection required to achieve full medial mobilization. Having identified the ureter, the inferior mesenteric artery may be divided. This technique is outlined in Chapter 4C. (The inferior mesenteric artery may also be preserved, if indicated, and this necessitates further dissection to identify the left colic artery for division and subsequent division of the sigmoid mesenteric vessels with preservation of the inferior mesenteric artery below.) The assistant now grasps the divided distal end of the inferior mesenteric artery and elevates this mesentery superiorly and laterally. The surgeon completes the medial mobilization on the underside of the descending colon and blunt dissection is carried out to reach the lateral abdominal wall, the lower pole of the spleen, and beyond the pelvic brim.

The assistant drops the cut end of the mesentery and may use a "Maryland" forceps to aid the surgeon in the lateral dissection. The surgeon uses the bowel grasper in his left hand and scissors in his right hand through the right-sided ports. The dissection is that of the lateral aspect of the paracolic gutter and commences at the sigmoid adhesions. The surgeon holds the distal sigmoid colon and traction applied to elevate the colon medially and toward the right upper quadrant. The incision is therefore at the lateral abdominal wall cephalad to the pelvic brim and into the virtual space created by the medial dissection. Once the surgeon connects the previous medial dissection and the new lateral incision, rapid progress may be made dissecting proximally along the paracolic gutter. The surgeon continues the dissection proximally to mobilize the colon from the paracolic gutter and once further progress is limited by instrument length the surgeon changes the scissors to the left lower quadrant and the bowel grasper to the right lower quadrant port site. This facilitates completion of the mobilization of the descending colon from lateral to medial and brings the surgeon as far as the splenic flexure.

MOBILIZATION AND DIVISION OF UPPER RECTUM, MESORECTUM, AND DESCENDING COLONIC MESENTERY

The surgeon should aim to keep the point of transection of the rectosigmoid junction in the upper rectum, just distal to the rectosigmoid junction. The surgeon remains on the patient's right side with the camera assistant on the surgeon's left. The patient remains in the Trendelenburg position. The rectosigmoid should be drawn anteriorly away from the pelvic brim to identify the fusion of the taenia coli on the antimesenteric border of the upper rectum. The lateral dissection may necessarily be continued into the upper rectum to free up the area for transection and similarly the right aspect of the mesorectum may also be dissected free from the peritoneal on the pelvic brim. This is facilitated on the left side by the assistant on the patient's left side using a Maryland forceps to provide tension laterally. The surgeon using the bowel grasper and scissors provides traction medially and divides the peritoneal reflection in between. The dissection of the peritoneal reflection on the right side of the rectum is easily divided using just the bowel grasper and scissors. Having mobilized the upper rectum, a point of transection should be chosen to permit a horizontal division of the rectum itself. The distal sigmoid is grasped and drawn superiorly and laterally by the assistant. The sigmoid mesentery is grasped with the surgeon's left-hand bowel grasper and a second bowel grasper is used to tease a passage between the under surface of the rectum and the superior rectal vessels. If the peritoneum has been opened on the left side already, the bowel grasper should work its way across and appear through this window. Care must be taken to avoid injury to the back wall of the rectum during this maneuver. Once this blunt dissection has been completed an ENDO GIA stapler is used to divide the rectum (see Figure 51.12). Two firings of the ENDO GIA are usually required. The mesorectum remaining after the rectum is transected may now be divided using cautery, the harmonic scalpel, LigaSure, or bipolar as preferred (see Figure 51.13).

The patient remains in the Trendelenburg position and dissection is carried out to ligate the descending colonic mesentery as far as the inferior mesenteric vein. The surgeon positioned at the patient's right side holds a bowel grasper through the right upper quadrant port and the LigaSure or harmonic scalpel through the right lower quadrant port. The camera assistant stands on the patient's right side. The assistant standing on the patient's left side uses a bowel grasper to elevate the proximal aspect of the descending colon and provide traction on the mesentery. The surgeon progressively divides the descending colonic mesentery. The key aspect of the dissection is the assistant providing enough traction to tent up the descending colon and allow progressive vessel ligation. The dissection is continued to the proximal aspect of the descending colon, which has already been mobilized from above.

CONFIRMATION OF COLONIC MOBILITY

The colon should now be completely free from all attachments. This needs to be confirmed before externalizing the specimen. The transverse colon should be elevated and a bowel grasper passed beneath the mesentery to confirm completion of the middle colic vessel division. The key areas to note are the splenic flexure and the hepatic flexure, as remnant attachments may be evident that were not apparent after the initial dissection. The mobility of the terminal ileum should also be checked and improved upon if necessary.

EXTERIORIZATION OF SPECIMEN AND PRESERVATION OF MESENTERIC ORIENTATION

The specimen is externalized through the umbilical port site. The divided end of the upper rectum is grasped with the right lower quadrant bowel grasper. The gas insufflation is turned off and the infraumbilical port removed. A 5-cm midline incision is made through the port site and umbilicus. The incision is deepened, and the linea alba and peritoneum are divided. A wound protector is used and the specimen delivered to the incision site. Using two Babcock forceps the colon is extracted. As the cecum is delivered, care must be taken to preserve the orientation of the terminal ileal mesentery. The terminal ileum is transected between two Kocher clamps and the ileal vascular arcade is assessed for good blood supply. The two marginal ileal mesenteric vessels are ligated between artery forceps. The purse-string suture of 0 polypropylene is inserted into the open end of the terminal ileum. The head of a 28-mm circular stapling gun is inserted and secured with a purse-string suture (see Figure 51.14). A laparoscopic Allis forceps is then inserted through the right lower quadrant port to grasp the obturator of the head of the gun. The orientation of the ileal mesentery is preserved as long as the Allis grasping forceps holds the head of the gun in the correct plane. It is therefore essential that this aspect of setting up the anastomosis is performed precisely. The Allis forceps maintains the hold on the head of the gun and the midline incision is then almost fully closed. The 10-mm infraumbilical port is reintroduced through this incompletely closed incision and the abdomen is reinsufflated.

**REINSUFFLA-
TION AND
ANASTOMOSIS**

The key elements in the completion of a laparoscopic ileorectal anastomosis are preservation of anastomotic integrity, prevention of torsion of the superior mesenteric arterial supply, and prevention of small bowel internal herniation. By delivering the terminal ileum back into the abdomen on a fixed Allis clamp, the alignment of the superior mesenteric artery should not be distorted. This needs to be assessed for anastomosis as the terminal ileum is laid down toward the pelvic brim. The mesentery of the small bowel needs to be traced back to the origin under the duodenum to confirm that there is no evidence of torsion. The small bowel should then be sequentially passed from one bowel clamp to another ("running the bowel") and laid in the left upper quadrant if possible. This is best facilitated with the patient remaining in the Trendelenburg position. Having determined that there is no herniation of the small bowel under the free edge of the ileal mesentery and that the superior mesenteric artery itself is not twisted, one may perform the ileorectal anastomosis (see Figure 51.15). The main body of the 28-mm circular stapler is introduced transanally and using a progressive rotation advanced to reach the transverse staple line of the transected rectal stump. The surgeon remains on the patient's right side with an Allis clamp in the left hand through the right upper quadrant and the second Allis clamp with the head of the gun attached through the right lower quadrant. A detailed account of this anastomotic technique is outlined in Chapter 4F. Once the head of the gun and the spike have been reconnected, a final check on the orientation of the mesentery and absence of internal herniation is performed. The gun is then approximated and fired. The circular "doughnuts" are tested and the anastomotic tension is assessed (see Figure 51.16). The bowel continuity is therefore reestablished with the ileorectal anastomosis and the anastomotic integrity is tested with subsequent insufflation under a pool of saline.

PORT CLOSURE

All port sites greater than 5 mm in size should be closed in a formal manner. In this case the right lower quadrant port site (12 mm), and if a 10-mm port was used in the left lower quadrant this also, requires closure. The details of formal port site closure are outlined in Chapter 4I.

J | PROCTOCOLECTOMY AND ILEAL POUCH ANAL ANASTOMOSIS

KEY STEPS

1. Patient positioning.

2. Insertion of ports: 10-mm umbilical Hasson technique; 12-mm right iliac fossa; 5-mm right upper quadrant; 5-mm left upper quadrant; 5- to 10-mm left iliac fossa.

3. Laparoscopic mobilization of right colon and terminal ileum.

4. Laparoscopic mobilization of transverse colon and take down of splenic flexure.

5. Division of middle colic vessels.

6. Laparoscopic mobilization of left colon.

7. Mobilization and division of upper rectum, mesorectum, and descending colonic mesentery.

8. Mobilization of rectum to anal canal.

9. Cross-stapling of rectum.

10. Exteriorization of colon with resection and division at terminal ileum.

11. Making of ileal pouch.

12. Return to laparoscopy and ileal pouch anal anastomosis.

13. Loop ileostomy.

The first steps of a laparoscopic ileal pouch procedure are identical to that of subtotal or total colectomy, and the text for this portion is identical to that of Chapter 51.

Two options exist for the ileal pouch procedure. Some surgeons perform a complete laparoscopic mobilization of the colon and rectum, divide the rectum laparoscopically, externalize the bowel through a short midline incision to remove the colon and make the ileal pouch, and reinsufflate the abdomen to complete the surgery. Other surgeons perform the colonic mobilization laparoscopically, and then perform a Pfannenstiel incision to complete mobilization of the rectum and making of the ileal pouch.

In this chapter and the video, we will describe the former approach, namely complete laparoscopic mobilization and laparoscopic reanastomosis. We use the latter approach selectively on men with a pelvis too narrow to complete dissection, or in whom a laparoscopic stapler cannot be placed successfully across the distal rectum.

Two videos accompany this chapter, one of the described approach and second of a "hybrid"-type procedure with laparoscopic colon mobilization and a Pfannenstiel incision for completion.

PATIENT POSITIONING

Correct positioning of the patient is of utmost importance when undertaking any laparoscopic resection but this is particularly true when mobilization of the transverse colon is necessitated. The patient undergoes general anaesthesia, with a Foley catheter and orogastric tube in place. The patient is placed on a beanbag with both arms tucked by the sides. The lower aspect of the beanbag should not encroach over the "break" in the operating table and the patient's buttocks should rest on this edge permitting easy access for a standard circular stapler to be used transanally to complete the ileorectal anastomosis. The patient's legs are placed in stirrups and in compression pneumatic stockings (see Figure 5J.1). The popliteal angle is maintained with slight flexion of the knee joint and the hip joint is supine with a slight extension and abduction if possible. Correct positioning of the lower limbs is essential as access to the transverse colon is significantly impeded if the quadriceps is bulky or if there is any hip flexion.

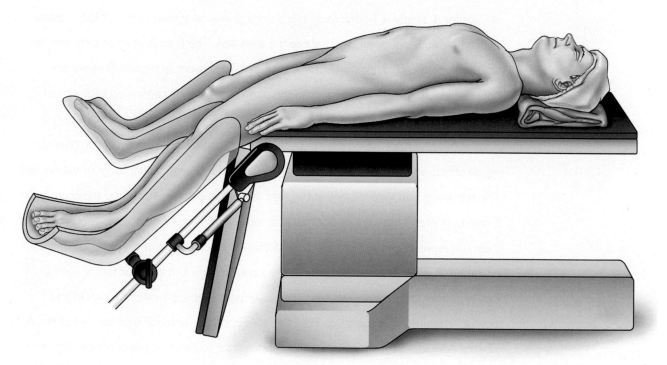

Figure 5J.1 The patient is positioned on the table in Dan Allen stirrups.

PORT INSERTION

There are five port sites used for a subtotal colectomy (see Figure 5J.2). The initial port site is an infraumbilical 10-mm port. This is the camera port and a good pneumatic seal is essential at this port site. A modified Hasson technique is used and is described in detail

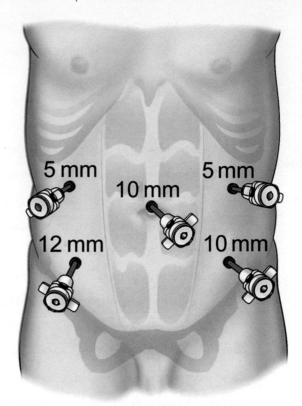

Figure 5J.2 Operating room setup for sigmoid procedures.

in Chapter 4. Briefly, a 1-cm infraumbilical vertical incision is made with a No. 11 blade and the incision is deepened to expose the linea alba. The linea is grasped between two Kocher forceps and an incision is made with a Mayo scissors to breach the linea and underlying peritoneum. The entry into the peritoneal cavity is confirmed with a blunt artery forceps (Kelly forceps), which should slide easily into the peritoneal cavity. A 0 polyglycolic acid purse-string suture is then used to secure the linea and aid in maintaining an effective seal. The 10-mm port is inserted and the pneumoperitoneum established. The remaining ports are located in the right and left upper quadrants and these are both 5-mm port sites. These are positioned at a comfortable hand's breath superiorly from their corresponding lower ports (12 to 15 cm). The positioning of these upper quadrant ports should avoid impedance of the lower costal margin and avoid potential "fencing" with their ipsilateral lower port. The lower port sites are located "1 inch in and 1 inch up" (medially and cephalad) from the corresponding anterior superior iliac spine. A 12-mm port site is used for the right lower quadrant to permit an endoscopic gastrointestinal stapler to be inserted for division of the rectum. A 5-mm left lower quadrant port is used to permit use of a harmonic ultrasonic instrument or a "LigaSure" bipolar instrument when ligating the ileocolic pedicle and middle colic vessels, as this has been our pratice due to the number of vessels being divided. This port site may necessarily be 10 mm in size if one uses a 10-mm harmonic scalpel or LigaSure device.

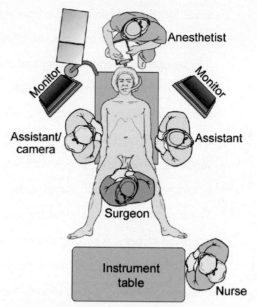

Figure 5J.3 Operating room setup for total colectomy with the surgeon positioned between the patient's legs.

INSTRUMENT POSITIONING AND LAPARO-SCOPIC ASSESSMENT

The case is dependent on having two monitors (see Figures 5J.3 and 5J.4). They are initially located on each side of the upper quadrants. The patient is prepped and draped to permit lateral access to the port sites. There should be two instrument-holding "quivers." These are attached, one on each side, on the lateral aspect of the patient's thighs. They contain two bowel-grasping forceps in each quiver and the dissecting electrocautery scissors, irrigation suction device, harmonic scalpel, or LigaSure instruments. The operating nurse should set up the instrument table opposite the patient's feet and allow sufficient

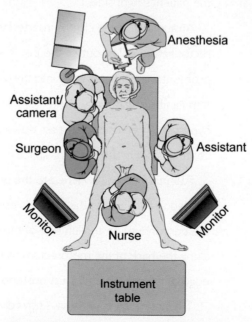

Figure 5J.4 Operating room setup for total colectomy with the surgeon positioned at the right side.

space for the surgeon to move from right or left to between the legs, as the case progresses. A 0-degree camera is used; however, a 30-degree lens or a flexible tip lens may be used with equal efficacy and may be particularly useful if there is a high splenic flexure or other anatomic variant. The initial assessment is a complete laparoscopy of the abdominal contents. Minor median adhesions obstructing assessment of the abdominal cavity should be dissected free and any unexpected pathology should be noted. The sequence of operating begins with mobilization of the right colon and terminal ileum in its entirety. The surgeon stands at the patient's left side at the level of the patient's hips. The surgical assistant stands at the surgeon's right side toward the patient's head and holds the camera. A second assistant is required in these cases and they in turn stand opposite the primary surgeon at the patient's right side, although he/she is generally needed only during mobilization of the transverse colon.

LAPAROSCOPIC MOBILIZATION OF THE COLON

Laparoscopic mobilization of the colon is as described in Chapter 5I

MOBILIZATION OF THE RECTUM DOWN TO THE ANAL CANAL

At this point in the procedure, the entire abdominal colon has been mobilized and the inferior mesenteric vessels have been divided. Attention is now turned to the pelvic dissection. The patient is in steep Trendelenburg position and rotated slightly to the right, with the small bowel reflected cranially. The surgeon and first assistant are standing at the patient's right side.

Atraumatic bowel clamps inserted through the left-sided ports are used to elevate the rectosigmoid colon out of the pelvis and away from the retroperitoneum and sacral promontory, to enable entry into the presacral space. The posterior aspect of the mesorectum can be identified and the mesorectal plane dissected with diathermy, preserving the hypogastric nerves as they pass down into the pelvis anterior to the sacrum. Dissection continues down the presacral space in this avascular plane toward the pelvic floor.

Attention is now switched to the peritoneum on the right side of the rectum. This is divided to the level of the seminal vesicles or rectovaginal septum. This is repeated on the peritoneum on the left side of the rectum. This facilitates further posterior dissection along the back of the mesorectum to the pelvic floor, to a level inferior to the lower edge of the mesorectum, just posterior to the anal canal (see Figure 5J.5).

The anterior peritoneum is now divided and dissection is continued down to the anal canal (see Figure 5J.6). An energy source such as the LigaSure is useful, as use of a simple shears with cautery often is difficult for the left side dissection as the instrument shorts onto the rectum. In those who have a particularly narrow or deep pelvis, perineal pressure can permit an extra couple of centimeters of dissection.

Once low in the pelvis, a bowel clamp may be placed through the left lower quadrant port and then the limbs are opened and the clamp nicely retracts the anterior structures away from the field of dissection.

An atraumatic bowel clamp through the left iliac fossa port is used to retract the peritoneum anterior to the rectum forward. The peritoneal dissection is continued from the free edge of the lateral peritoneal dissection, anteriorly. Lateral dissection is continued on both sides of the rectum and is extended anterior to the rectum, posterior to Denonvillier's fascia, separating the posterior vaginal wall from the anterior wall of the rectum (in a female patient) or down to the level of the prostate (in a male patient). The difficulty of dissection will vary depending on the body habitus of the patient, the diameter of the pelvis, and the size of the tumor. Rectal mobilization can be difficult to perform laparoscopically, on occasion. In some cases, it may need to be completed in an open manner through a small Pfannenstiel incision.

RECTAL DIVISION

A roticulating endoscopic stapler may be used laparoscopically to divide the muscle tube of the anorectal junction below the level of the mesorectum. The stapler is inserted through the right lower quadrant incision, and two firings of the stapler are usually required to divide the rectum. Traction of the midrectum to the left permits the stapler to be placed perpendicularly across the bowel at this level (see Figure 5J.7). There is no residual mesorectum to divide at this level. Digital examination is performed to confirm the location of the distal staple line after placement of the stapler and before division of the bowel, aiming to have the transverse staple line approximately 1.5 cm above the dentate line, so that the final pouch—anal anastomosis comes to lie 1 cm from the dentate line (see Figure 5J.8).

It is sometimes impossible to divide the rectum laparoscopically as the angulation of the endovascular stapler is limited to 45 degrees, necessitating open division of the rectum. For this reason, it is very useful to employ a stapler with as short a distance between the tip and the angle of reticulation. In some patients, getting an assistant to push up on the perineum with their hand may lift the pelvic floor enough to get the first cartridge of the stapler low enough. In some cases, placing a suprapubic port allows easier access with the stapler to allow division of the rectum.

Some patients are either too obese or have a very narrow pelvis or a long anal canal, and the stapler cannot be passed low enough. Two options exist. One is to perform a transanal intersphincteric dissection, remove the specimen, and then perform a hand-sewn coloanal anastomosis. The second is to perform a short Pfannenstiel incision, which allows a linear 30-mm stapler to be positioned and the rectum divided.

CONFIRMATION OF COLONIC MOBILITY

The colon and rectum should now be completely free from all attachments. This needs to be confirmed before externalizing the specimen. The transverse colon should be elevated and a bowel grasper passed beneath the mesentery to confirm completion of the middle colic vessel division. The key areas to note are the splenic flexure and the hepatic flexure as remnant attachments may be evident that were not apparent after initial dissection. The mobility of the terminal ileum should also be checked and improved upon if necessary, so that there will be easy reach for ileoanal anastomosis.

EXTERIORIZATION OF SPECIMEN AND PRESERVATION OF MESENTERIC ORIENTATION

The specimen is externalized through an incision at the umbilical port site. The divided end of the upper rectum is grasped with the right lower quadrant bowel grasper. The gas insufflation is turned off and the infraumbilical port is removed. A 4- to 5-cm midline incision is made through the port site and umbilicus. The incision is deepened and linea alba and peritoneum are divided. Using two Babcock forceps the colon is extracted. The terminal ileum is transected between two Kocher clamps and the ileal vascular arcade assessed for good blood supply. The two marginal ileal mesenteric vessels are ligated between artery forceps.

The apex of the ileal pouch is chosen and an enterotomy is performed. A 15- to 20-cm ileal pouch is made with multiple firings of a 100-mm or 80-mm GIA stapler through the enterotomy. The tip of the J-pouch is closed with a further cartridge, and the pouch distended with saline and checked for integrity. The inside of the pouch is inspected to make sure there are no bleeding vessels. A purse-string suture of 0 polypropylene is inserted into the open end of the terminal ileum. The head of a 28-mm circular stapling gun is inserted and secured (see Figure 5J.9). The pouch is returned to the abdomen and the midline incision is partially closed. The 10-mm port is reintroduced through this incompletely closed incision and the abdomen is reinsufflated.

REINSUFFLATION AND ANASTOMOSIS

The key elements in the completion of a laparoscopic ileoanal anastomosis are preservation of anastomotic integrity, prevention of torsion of the superior mesenteric arterial supply, and prevention of small bowel internal herniation. Orientation of the pouch mesentery is assessed as the terminal ileum is laid down toward the pelvic brim for anastomosis. The mesentery of the small bowel needs to be traced back to the origin under the duodenum to confirm orientation.

Having determined that there is no herniation of the small bowel under the free edge of the ileal mesentery and that the superior mesenteric artery itself is not twisted, one may perform the pouch–anal anastomosis. The instruments in the left side ports may be used for anterior retraction of the bladder and prostate or vagina, to allow visualization of the rectal stump. The main body of the 28-mm circular stapler is cautiously introduced transanally and using a progressive rotation advanced to reach the transverse staple line (see Figure 5J.10) of the transected anorectal stump.

The surgeon remains on the patient's right side with an Allis clamp in the left hand through the right upper quadrant and the second Allis clamp with the head of the gun attached through the right lower quadrant (see Figure 5J.11). Once the head of the gun and the spike have been reconnected, a final check of the orientation of the mesentery and absence of internal herniation is performed (see Figure 5J.12). The gun is then approximated and fired. The circular "doughnuts" are tested and anastomotic tension is assessed. Anastomotic integrity is tested with subsequent insufflation under a pool of saline (see Figure 5J.13).

PORT CLOSURE

All port sites greater than 5 mm in size should be closed in a formal manner. In this case, the right lower quadrant port site (12 mm) and if a 10-mm port was used in the left lower quadrant, this also requires closure.

LOOP ILEOSTOMY

In our practice, ileoanal anastomoses are almost always diverted with a loop ileostomy. This is no different in our open or laparoscopic procedures. Having completed the above procedure and closed all ports, a suitable piece of ileum is chosen for loop ileostomy at the preoperatively marked site. The abdomen is desufflated and the ileostomy performed through the small midline incision. The fascia is closed, and the skin closed with subcuticular stitches.

STOMA FORMATION

LOOP SIGMOID COLOSTOMY

KEY STEPS

1. Insertion of ports: 10-mm umbilical Hasson technique; 5-mm right iliac fossa; 5-mm right upper quadrant.

2. Patient turned to Trendelenburg position.

3. Laparoscopic assessment, and small bowel and omentum moved toward right upper quadrant.

4. Division of lateral attachments of sigmoid colon.

5. Formation of trephine colostomy site in left iliac fossa at site marked by enterostomal therapist.

6. Delivery of sigmoid through trephine and maturation of loop stoma.

7. Closure of umbilical port site.

PATIENT POSITIONING

The patient is placed supine on the operating table, on a beanbag. After induction of general anesthesia and insertion of an oro-gastric tube and Foley catheter, the legs are placed in Dan Allen or Yellowfin stirrups (see Figure 5K.1). The arms are tucked at the patient's side and the beanbag is aspirated. The abdomen is prepared with antiseptic solution and draped routinely (see Chapter 4).

INSTRUMENT POSITIONING

The primary monitor is placed on the left side of the patient at the level of the hip (see Figure 5K.2). The operating nurse's instrument table is placed between the patient's legs. There should be sufficient space to allow the surgeon to move from either side of the patient to between the patient's legs, if necessary. The primary operating surgeon stands at the right side of the patient with the assistant standing on the patient's left, and moving to the right side, caudad to the surgeon once ports have been inserted. A 0-degree camera lens is used.

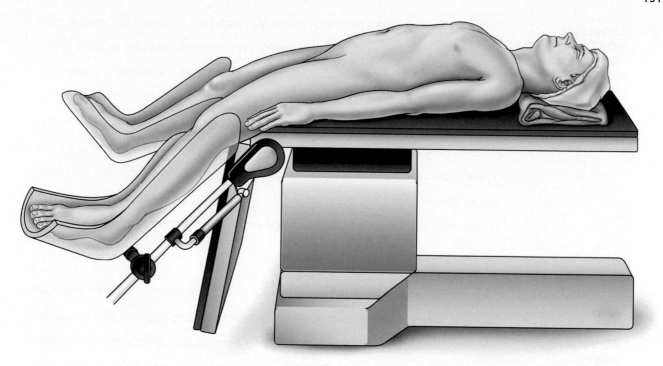

Figure 5K.1 The patient is positioned on the table in Dan Allen stirrups.

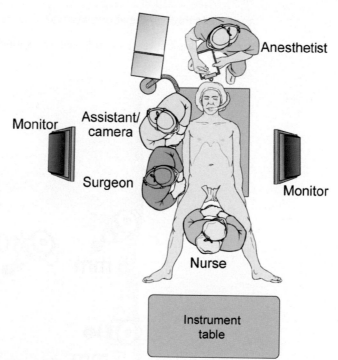

Figure 5K.2 Operating room setup for loop colostomy with the surgeon positioned on the right side.

UMBILICAL PORT INSERTION

This is performed using a modified Hasson approach (see Chapter 4). A vertical 1-cm subumbilical incision is made. This is deepened down to the linea alba, which is then grasped on each side of the midline using Kocher clamps. A scalpel (No. 15 blade) is used to open the fascia between the Kocher clamps and a Kelly forceps is used to open the peritoneum bluntly. It is important to keep this opening small (<1 cm) to minimize air leaks. Having confirmed entry into the peritoneal cavity, a purse-string suture of 0 polyglycolic acid is placed around the subumbilical fascial defect (umbilical port site) and a Rommel tourniquet is applied. A 10-mm reusable port is inserted through this port site allowing the abdomen to be insufflated with CO_2 to a pressure of 12 mm Hg.

LAPAROSCOPY AND INSERTION OF REMAINING PORTS

The camera is inserted into the abdomen and an initial laparoscopy is performed, carefully evaluating the liver, small bowel, and peritoneal surfaces. A 5-mm port is inserted in the right lower quadrant approximately 2 to 3 cm medial and superior to the anterior superior iliac spine (see Figure 5K.3). This is carefully inserted lateral to the inferior epigastric vessels, paying attention to keep the tract of the port going as perpendicular as possible through the abdominal wall. A 5-mm port is then inserted through the right upper quadrant at least a hand's breadth superior to the lower quadrant port.

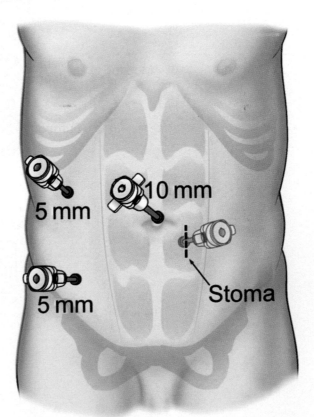

Figure 5K.3 Port setup for colostomy.

DEFINITIVE LAPARO-SCOPIC SETUP

The assistant now moves to the patient's right side, standing caudad to the surgeon. The patient is rotated with the left side up and right side down, to approximately 15 to 20 degrees tilt, and often as far as the table can go. This helps to move the small bowel over to the right side of the abdomen. The patient is then placed in the Trendelenburg position. This again helps gravitational migration of the small bowel away from the surgical field. The surgeon then inserts two atraumatic bowel clamps through the two right-sided abdominal ports. The greater omentum is reflected over the transverse colon so that it comes to lie on the stomach. If there is no space in the upper part of the abdomen, one must confirm that the orogastric tube is adequately decompressing the stomach.

DIVISION OF LATERAL ATTACH-MENTS OF SIGMOID COLON

The sigmoid colon is grasped by the surgeon using two atraumatic bowel clamps to assess its mobility. If the colon is not easily raised toward the abdominal wall without tension, it is necessary to mobilize the lateral attachments of the sigmoid colon. The sigmoid colon is mobilized by dividing the lateral attachments along the white line of Toldt. It is usually necessary to mobilize only the colon such that the sigmoid colon can reach the anterior abdominal wall. Once the pneumoperitoneum is released, the colon will then be able to be delivered without tension. Depending on how mobile the descending colon and sigmoid are, a variable amount of mobilization needs to be performed.

FORMATION OF TREPHINE LEFT ILIAC FOSSA COLOSTOMY

A colostomy trephine is made in the left iliac fossa at a site that has been marked by an enterostomal therapist before surgery. A skin disk is excised, a longitudinal incision is made in the anterior rectus sheath, and the left rectus muscle is split. The peritoneum is held with two hemostats and incised. The sigmoid colon is delivered to the trephine, grasped with Babcock forceps, and delivered through the trephine. A short plastic stoma rod is passed between the mesentery and bowel to support the colon.

PORT SITE CLOSURE AND STOMA MATURATION

The umbilical port site is closed using the previously inserted purse-string suture, and skin incisions are closed. The loop of the sigmoid colon is incised and the loop colostomy matured using 3/0 chromic catgut.

L | LOOP ILEOSTOMY

KEY STEPS

1. Insertion of ports: 10-mm umbilical Hasson technique; 5-mm left iliac fossa; optional 5-mm left upper quadrant.

2. Patient turned to Trendelenburg position.

3. Laparoscopic assessment, and small bowel and omentum moved toward left upper quadrant.

4. Assessment of reach of terminal ileum.

5. Optional division of lateral attachments of cecum and terminal ileum.

6. Formation of trephine site in right iliac fossa at site marked by enterostomal therapist.

7. Delivery of terminal ileum through trephine and maturation of loop stoma.

8. Closure of umbilical port site.

PATIENT POSITIONING

The patient is placed supine on the operating table, on a beanbag. After induction of general anesthesia and insertion of an oral gastric tube and Foley catheter, the legs are placed in Dan Allen or Yellowfin stirrups (see Figure 5L.1). The arms are tucked at the patient's side and the beanbag is aspirated. The abdomen is prepared with antiseptic solution and draped routinely (see Chapter 4).

INSTRUMENT POSITIONING

The primary monitor is placed on the right side of the patient at the level of the hip (see Figure 5L.2). The operating nurse's instrument table is placed between the patient's legs. There should be sufficient space to allow the surgeon to move from either side of the patient to between the patient's legs, if necessary. The primary operating surgeon stands at the left side of the patient with the assistant standing at the patient's right, and moving to the left side, caudad to the surgeon once ports have been inserted. A 0-degree camera lens is used.

UMBILICAL PORT INSERTION

This is performed using a modified Hasson approach (see Chapter 4). A vertical 1-cm subumbilical incision is made. This is deepened down to the linea alba, which is then grasped on each side of the midline using Kocher clamps. A scalpel (No. 15 blade) is

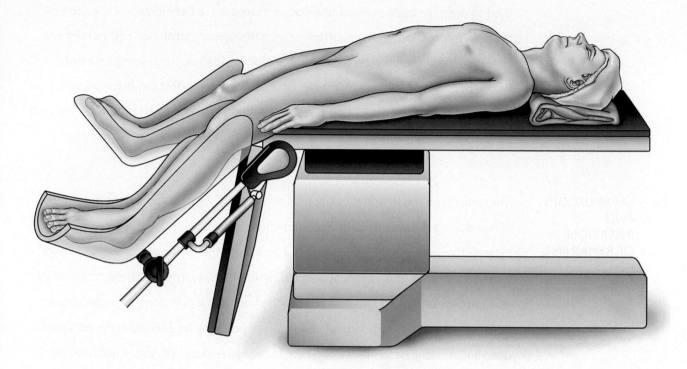

Figure 5L.1 The patient is positioned on the table in Dan Allen stirrups.

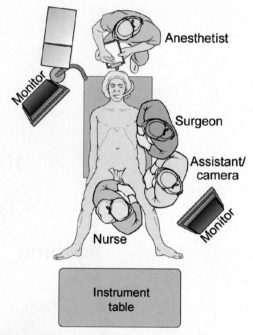

Figure 5L.2 Operating room setup for right side procedures.

used to open the fascia between the Kocher clamps and a Kelly forceps is used to open the peritoneum bluntly. It is important to keep this opening small (<1 cm) to minimize air leaks. Having confirmed entry into the peritoneal cavity, a purse-string suture of 0 polyglycolic acid is placed around the subumbilical fascial defect (umbilical port site) and a Rommel tourniquet is applied. A 10-mm reusable port is inserted through this port site allowing the abdomen to be insufflated with CO_2 to a pressure of 12 mm Hg.

LAPAROSCOPY AND INSERTION OF REMAINING PORTS

The camera is inserted into the abdomen and an initial laparoscopy is performed, carefully evaluating the liver, small bowel, and peritoneal surfaces. A 5-mm port is inserted in the left lower quadrant approximately 2 to 3 cm medial and superior to the anterior superior iliac spine (see Figures 5L.3 and 5L.4). It is carefully inserted lateral to the inferior epigastric vessels, paying attention to keep the tract of the port going as perpendicular as possible through the abdominal wall. A 5-mm port may be inserted in the left upper quadrant at least a hand's breath superior to the lower quadrant port, if necessary, to perform some dissection to mobilize the terminal ileum.

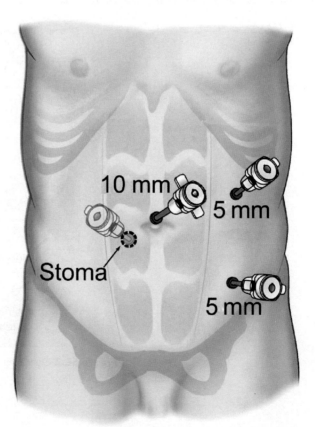

Figure 5L.3 Port setup for ileostomy.

DEFINITIVE LAPARO-SCOPIC SETUP

The assistant now moves to the patient's left side, standing caudad to the surgeon. The patient is rotated with the right side up and left side down, to approximately 15 to 20 degrees tilt. This helps to move the small bowel over to the left side of the abdomen. The patient is then placed in the Trendelenburg position. This again helps gravitational migration of the small bowel away from the surgical field. The surgeon then inserts one or two atraumatic bowel clamps through the left-sided abdominal port(s). The greater omentum is reflected over the transverse colon so that it comes to lie on the stomach. If there is no space in the upper part of the abdomen, one must confirm that the orogastric tube is adequately decompressing the stomach.

DIVISION OF LATERAL ATTACH-MENTS OF CECUM AND TERMINAL ILEUM

The terminal ileum is grasped by the surgeon using atraumatic bowel clamps to assess its mobility (see Figure 5L.5). If the bowel is not easily raised toward the abdominal wall without tension, it is necessary to mobilize the lateral attachments of the cecum and sometimes the posterior attachments of the terminal ileum. The cecum is mobilized by dividing the lateral attachments along the white line of Toldt (see Figure 5L.6). It is usually necessary to mobilize only the colon such that the terminal ileum can reach the anterior abdominal wall. Once the pneumoperitoneum is released, the intestine will then be able to be delivered without tension. Depending on how mobile the terminal ileum and cecum are, a variable amount of mobilization needs to be performed.

FORMATION OF TREPHINE FOR RIGHT LOWER QUADRANT ILEOSTOMY

An ileostomy trephine is made in the right lower quadrant at a site that has been marked by an enterostomal therapist before surgery. A skin disk is excised, a longitudinal incision is made in the anterior rectus sheath, and the left rectus muscle is split. The peritoneum is held with two hemostats and incised. The terminal ileum is brought to the trephine, grasped with Babcock forceps, and delivered through the trephine. A short plastic stoma rod is passed between the mesentery and the bowel to support the intestine. The laproscope is then reinserted and orientation of the ileostomy is confirmed (see Figures 5L.7 and 5L.8).

PORT SITE CLOSURE AND STOMA MATURATION

The umbilical port site is closed using the previously inserted purse-string suture, and skin incisions are closed. The loop of sigmoid colon is incised and the loop colostomy is matured using 3/0 chromic catgut.

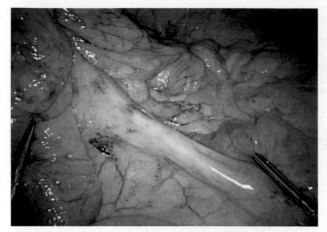

Figure 5A.4 The ileocolic pedicle and the duodenum.

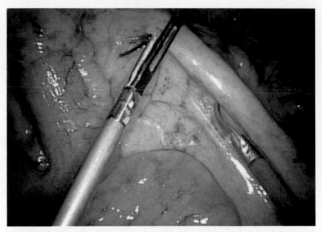

Figure 5A.5 Dissecting the ileocolic pedicle.

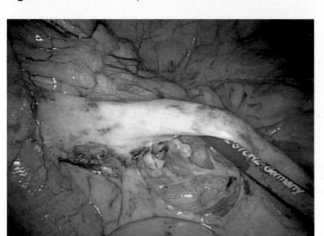

Figure 5A.6 Isolating the ileocolic pedicle.

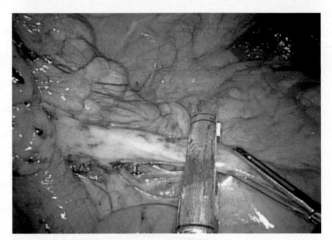

Figure 5A.7 Dividing the ileocolic pedicle.

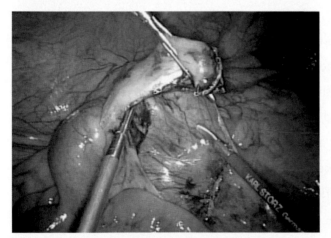

Figure 5A.8 Commencing the medial dissection of the ascending colon.

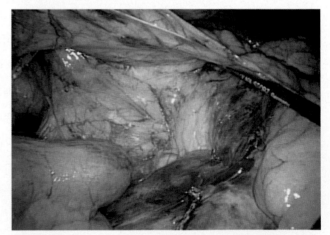

Figure 5A.9 Continuing the medial dissection of the ascending colon.

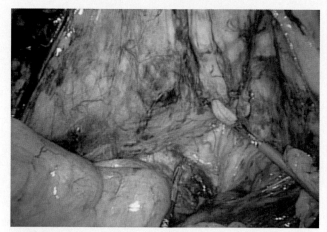

Figure 5A.10 Completing the medial (retroperitoneal) mobilization of the ascending colon.

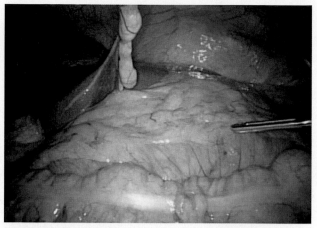

Figure 5A.11 Identifying the fusion line of omentum and transverse colon.

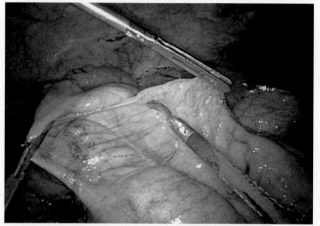

Figure 5A.12 Starting to take down the hepatic flexure.

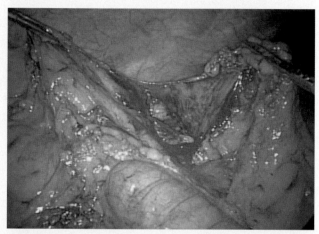

Figure 5A.13 Developing the plane behind the hepatic flexure.

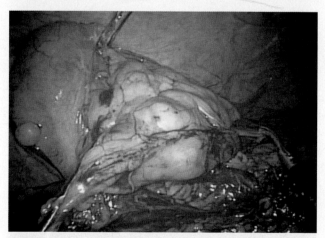

Figure 5A.14 Continuing the lateral mobilization of the hepatic flexure and the ascending colon.

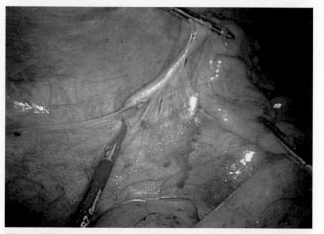

Figure 5A.15 Mobilizing the appendix and the cecum.

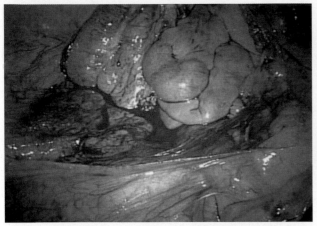

Figure 5A.16 Completing mobilization of the cecum and the small bowel mesentery.

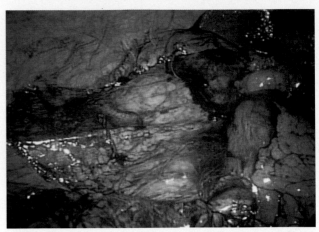

Figure 5A.17 After complete mobilization the right colon is rotated.

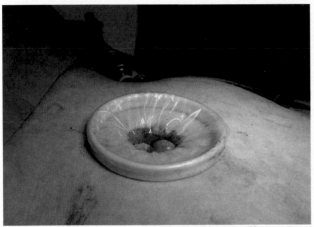

Figure 5A.18 The right colon is exteriorized through a small wound using a wound protector.

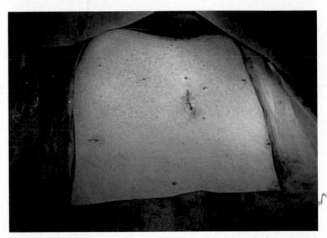

Figure 5A.19 The incisions are closed with subcuticular sutures.

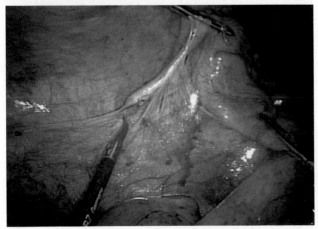

Figure 5B.4 Identifying the fusion line of omentum and transverse colon.

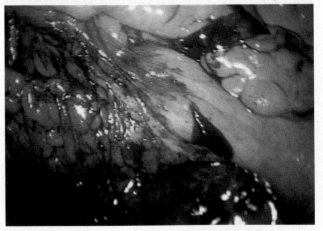

Figure 5B.5 The omentum is elevated and dissected off the transverse colon.

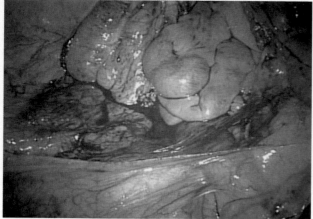

Figure 5B.6 The hepatic flexure is then mobilized.

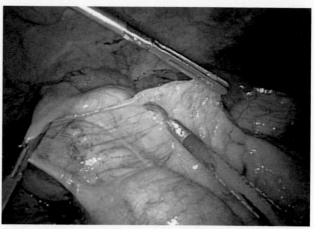

Figure 5B.7 The plane behind the hepatic flexure is developed.

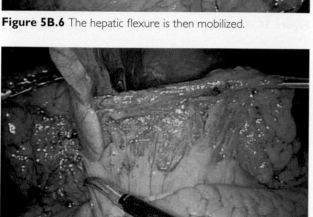

Figure 5B.8 Lateral mobilization of the hepatic flexure and the ascending colon.

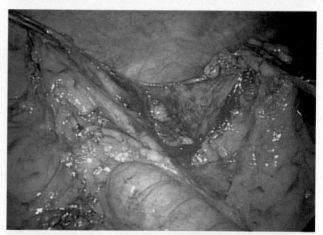

Figure 5B.9 Mobilizing the appendix and the cecum.

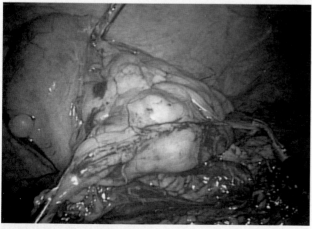

Figure 5B.10 The inflamed terminal ileal mesentery is dissected off the retroperitoneum.

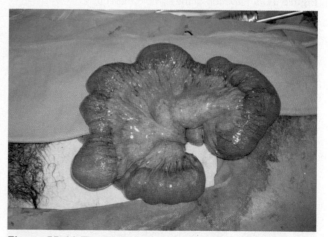

Figure 5B.11 The terminal ileum and the distal small bowel can be exteriorized through a short midline wound.

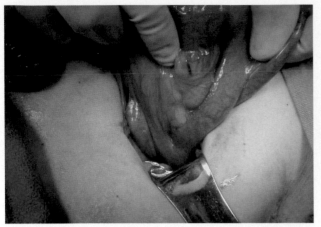

Figure 5B.12 The small bowel can be palpated throughout its length by sequential exteriorization, palpating up the duodenojejunal flexure.

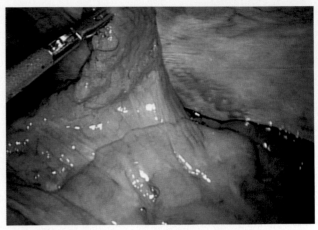

Figure 5C.4 The omentum is reflected in a cephalad direction over the stomach.

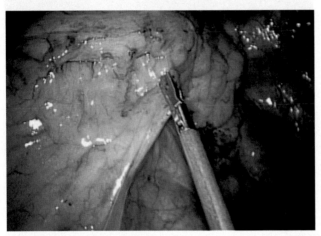

Figure 5C.5 Elevation of the sigmoid mesentery.

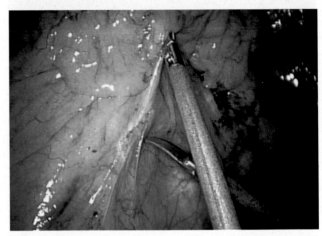

Figure 5C.6 Incising the peritoneum to define the inferior mesenteric vessels.

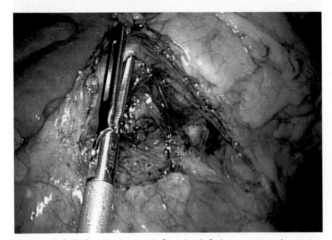

Figure 5C.7 Continuing to define the inferior mesenteric artery for low ligation.

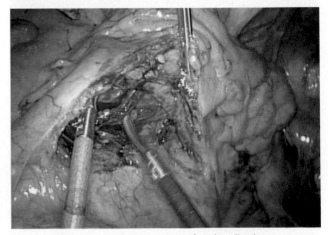

Figure 5C.8 Identifying the ureter before low ligation.

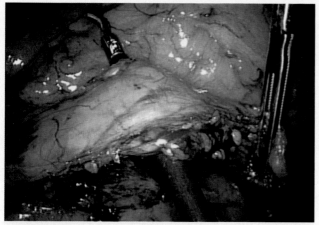

Figure 5C.9 Preparing the inferior mesenteric artery for division.

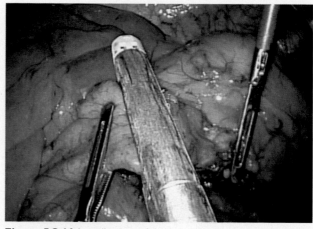

Figure 5C.10 Low ligation of the inferior mesenteric artery.

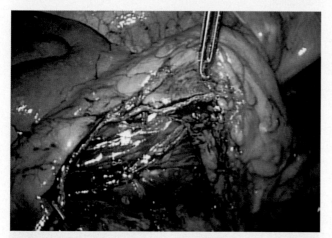

Figure 5C.11 Medial retroperitoneal dissection under the mesentery.

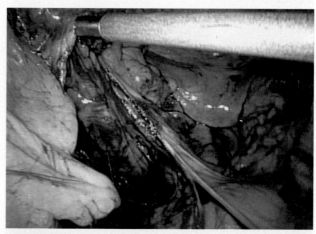

Figure 5C.12 The right side of the mesorectum is partially mobilized.

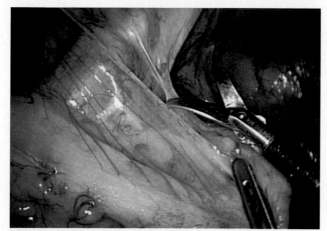

Figure 5C.13 The lateral attachments of the rectosigmoid are mobilized.

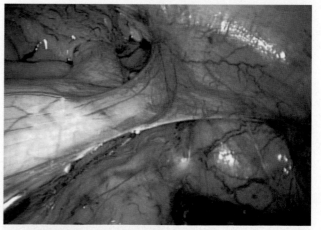

Figure 5C.14 The lateral attachments of the descending colon are mobilized up to the splenic flexure.

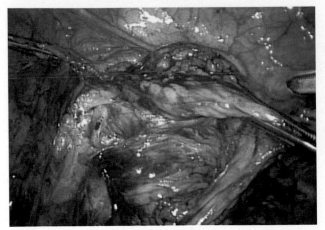

Figure 5C.15 The left lateral attachments of the mesorectum are mobilized.

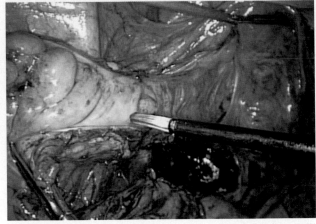

Figure 5C.16 The rectosigmoid junction is defined for rectal transection.

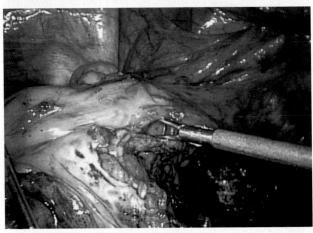

Figure 5C.17 A plane is developed between the rectum and mesorectum.

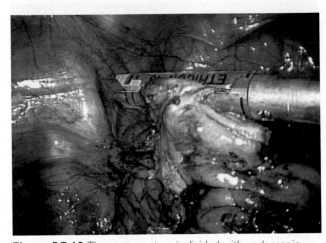

Figure 5C.18 The upper rectum is divided with endoscopic staplers.

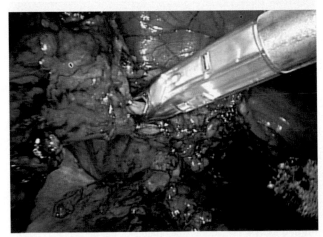

Figure 5C.19 The mesorectum is then divided using clips and cautery.

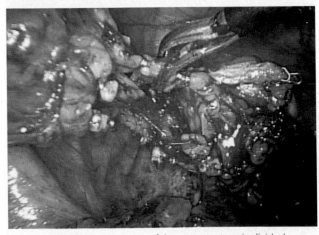

Figure 5C.20 The final part of the mesorectum is divided.

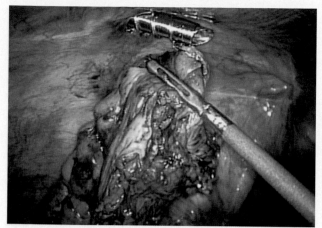

Figure 5C.21 Adequate mobilization of the sigmoid is confirmed.

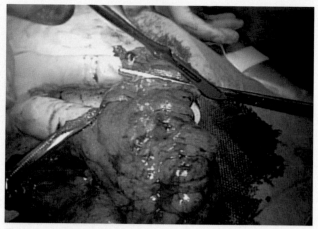

Figure 5C.22 The bowel is divided after exteriorization through a left lower quadrant incision.

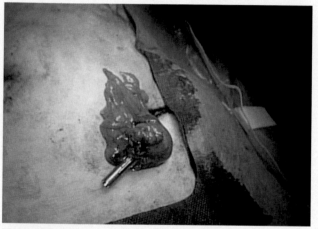

Figure 5C.23 The anvil is placed in the proximal bowel before closing the fascia.

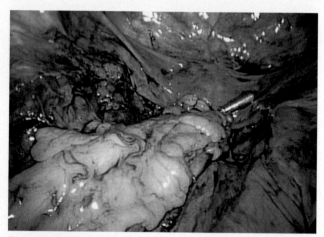

Figure 5C.24 Adequate reach of the proximal bowel is checked to permit a tension-free anastomosis.

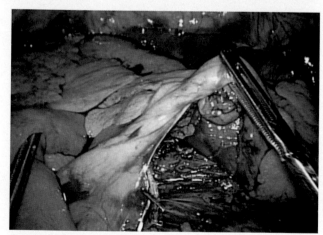

Figure 5C.25 The orientation of the mesentery is confirmed.

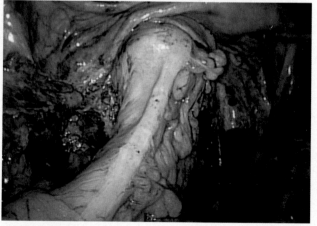

Figure 5C.26 The anastomosis is performed.

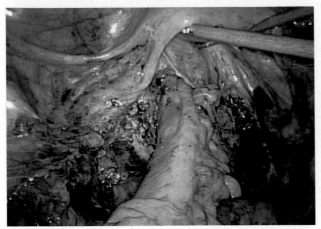

Figure 5C.27 The anastomosis lies in the pelvis below the pelvic brim.

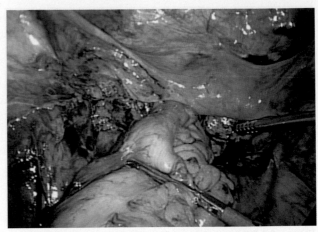

Figure 5C.28 The anastomosis is tested by air distension under water.

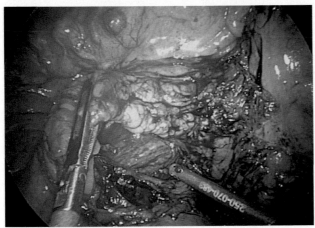

Figure 5D.4 The inferior mesenteric vessels are defined, carefully protecting the autonomic nerves and the ureter.

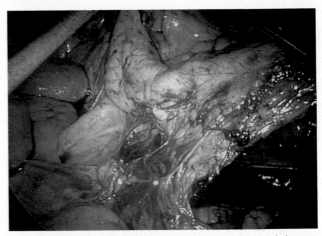

Figure 5D.5 The origin of the inferior mesenteric vessels is carefully defined.

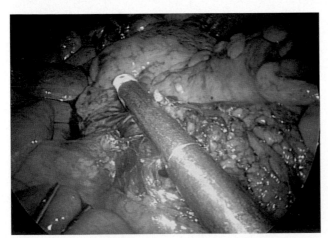

Figure 5D.6 The inferior mesenteric artery is divided with a high ligation.

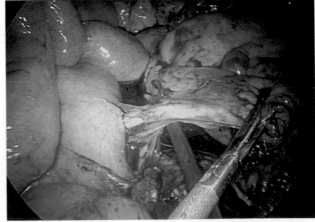

Figure 5D.7 The inferior mesenteric vein is divided high, close to the duodenojejunal flexure and tail of pancreas.

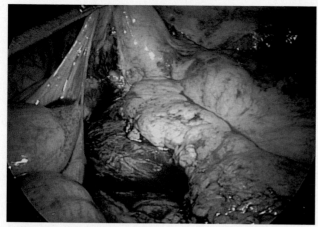

Figure 5D.8 Having divided the inferior mesenteric vessels, the reach of the descending colon is optimized for a coloanal anastomosis.

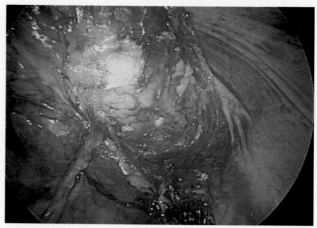

Figure 5D.9 The mesorectum is mobilized carefully protecting the autonomic nerves.

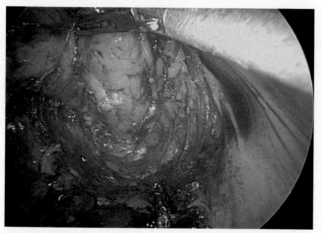

Figure 5D.10 The dissection continues into the pelvis, preserving the presacral fascia.

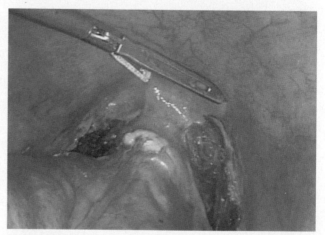

Figure 5D.11 The right side of the mesorectum is mobilized.

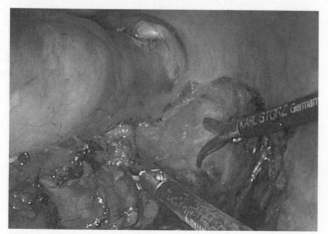

Figure 5D.12 The left side of the mesorectum is mobilized.

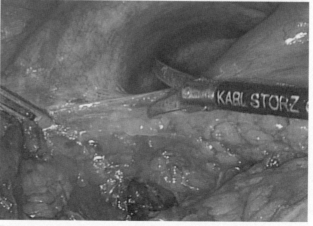

Figure 5D.13 An anterior mobilization is then performed.

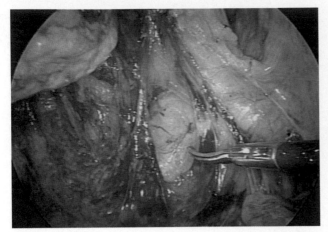

Figure 5D.14 The posterior dissection is then completed.

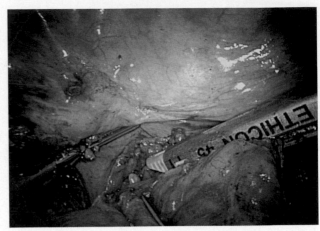

Figure 5D.15 A stapler is placed 5 cm distal to an upper rectal cancer or at the anal canal, after performing a total mesorectal dissection.

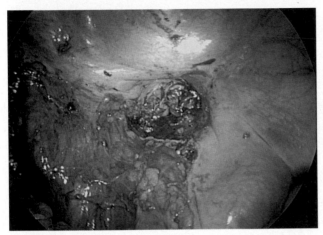

Figure 5D.16 The rectum is divided.

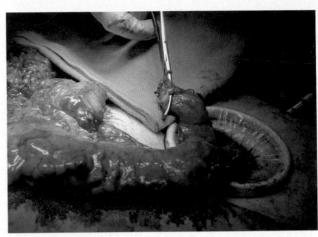

Figure 5D.17 The specimen is extracted through the left lower quadrant incision using a wound protector.

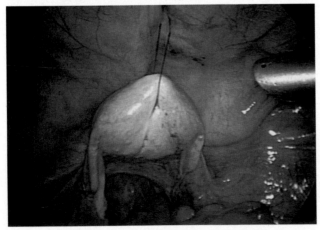

Figure 5E.4 The uterus is hitched out of the way in female patients.

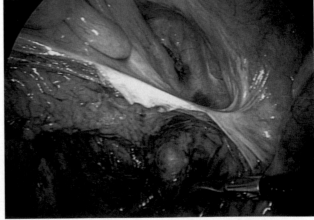

Figure 5E.5 Having divided the inferior mesenteric vessels, the posterior surface of the mesorectum is mobilized.

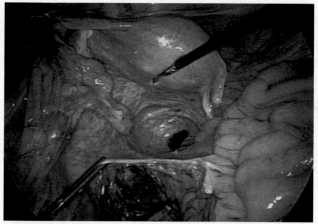

Figure 5E.6 The left side of the mesorectum is mobilized.

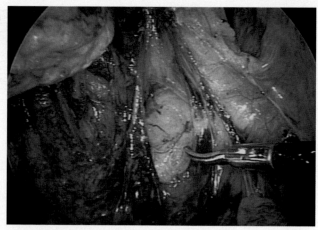

Figure 5E.7 This allows deeper access to the pelvis to complete the posterior mobilization down to the anal canal.

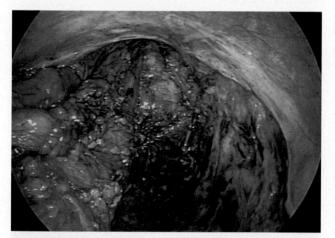

Figure 5E.8 The right side mobilization is completed.

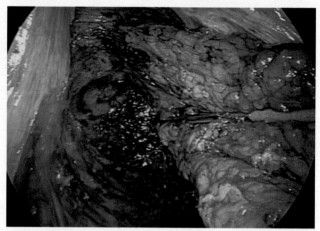

Figure 5E.9 The left side of the mesorectum is then completely mobilized.

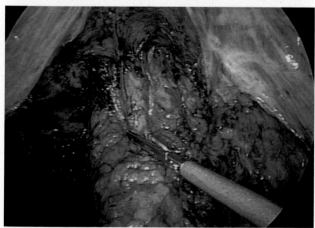

Figure 5E.10 The final anterior attachments are then divided, completing the mesorectal mobilization.

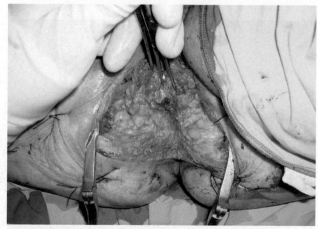

Figure 5E.11 The lowest part of the dissection is performed transperineally.

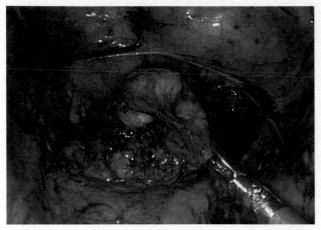

Figure 5F.3 Adhesions are lysed to allow identification of the rectal stump.

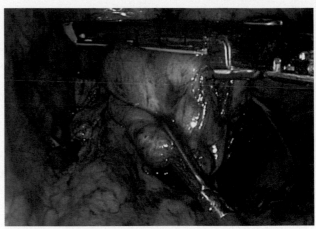

Figure 5F.4 If there is any distal sigmoid colon remaining, this is resected to allow transection immediately distal to the rectosigmoid junction.

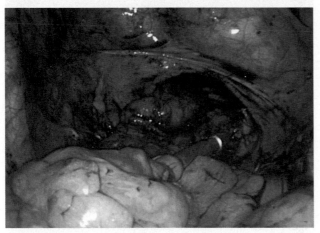

Figure 5F.5 The proximal colon is mobilized so that the colon easily reaches into the pelvis.

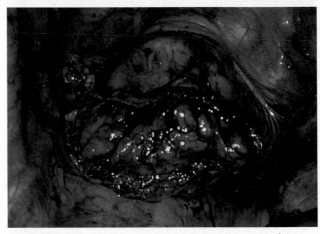

Figure 5F.6 The staple gun is inserted up to the apex of the rectal stump.

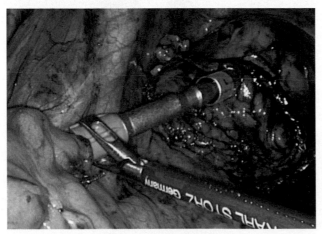

Figure 5F.7 The anastomosis is performed.

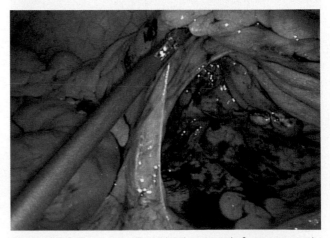

Figure 5F.8 The descending colon is assessed after anastomosis to ensure that there is no tension present.

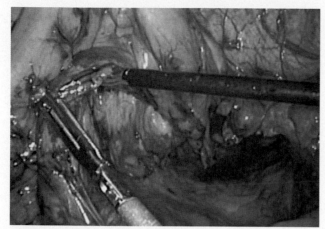

Figure 5H.4 The inferior mesenteric artery is defined and mobilized, carefully protecting the presacral autonomic nerves and ureters.

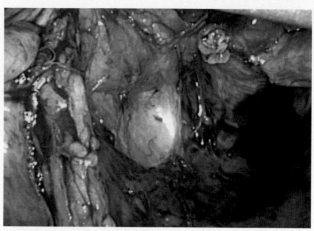

Figure 5H.5 A presacral mobilization of the rectum and mesorectum is performed.

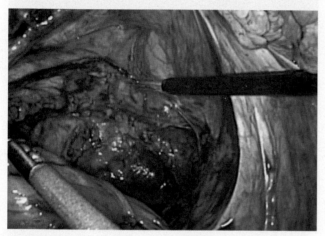

Figure 5H.6 The lateral attachments of the rectum are mobilized, preserving the lateral ligaments unless they require to be divided to completely reduce the prolapse.

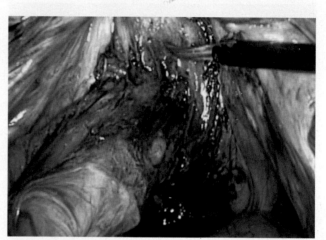

Figure 5H.7 The anterior aspect of the rectum is mobilized only if necessary to have a complete, tension-free reduction of the prolapse.

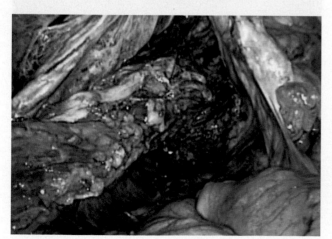

Figure 5H.8 The prolapse is completely reduced and the pelvis is checked for hemostasis.

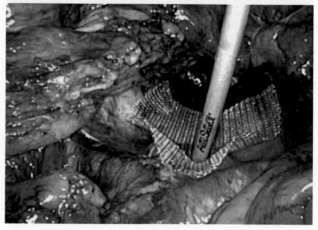

Figure 5H.9 The mesh is inserted and fixed to the sacral promontory in the midline.

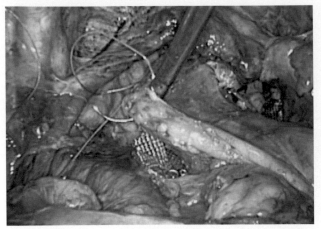

Figure 5H.10 The left side of the mesorectum is fixed to the mesh.

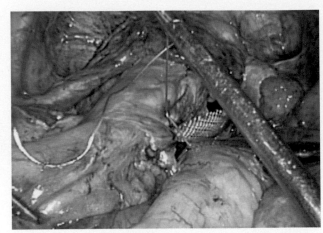

Figure 5H.11 The right side of the mesorectum is then fixed to the mesh.

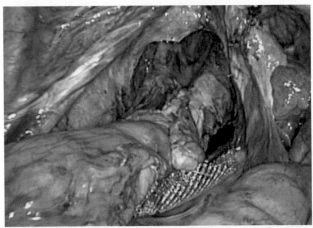

Figure 5H.12 The rectum can be seen to be completely reduced and suspended to the sacral promontory by the mesh.

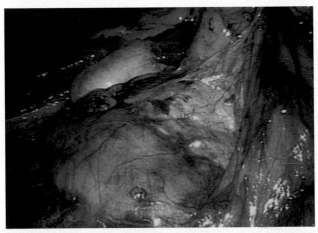

Figure 5I.5 The hepatic flexure and right colon are mobilized exposing the pancreas and duodenum.

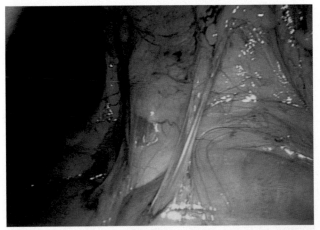

Figure 5I.6 The greater omentum is elevated and distracted from the transverse colon.

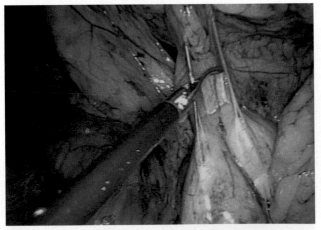

Figure 5I.7 The greater omentum is dissected off the transverse colon, staying in the avascular plane between the two structures.

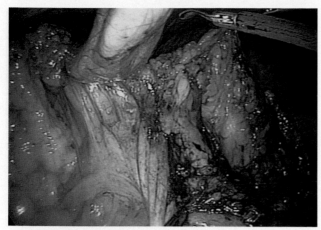

Figure 51.8 The dissection continues until the transverse colon has been completely mobilized.

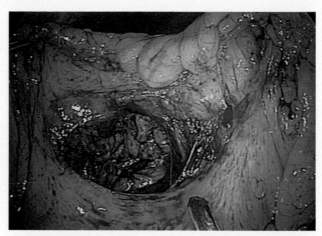

Figure 51.9 The transverse colon is then elevated, displaying the windows to each side of the middle colic vessels.

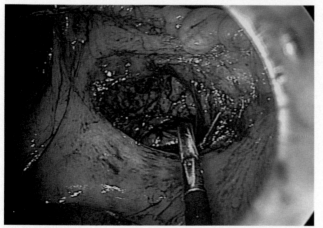

Figure 51.10 The mesocolic vessels are carefully defined before division with clip stapler of an alternative energy source.

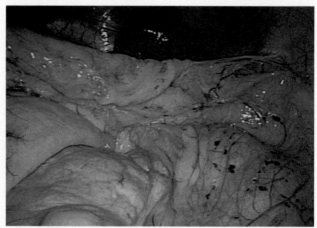

Figure 51.11 The splenic flexure and left colon are then mobilized, exposing the pancreas and duodenum.

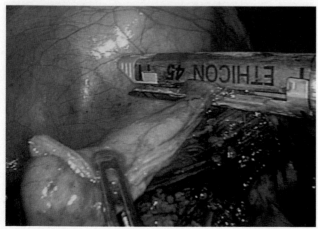

Figure 51.12 The rectosigmoid junction is divided with staple cartridges.

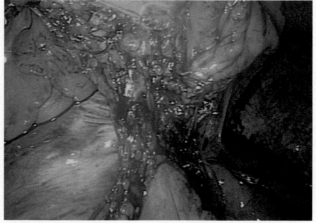

Figure 51.13 The mesentery of the sigmoid is divided, completing mobilization of the intraabdominal colon.

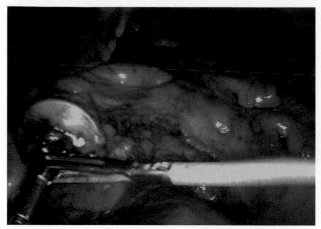

Figure 51.14 After resecting the bowel extracorporeally and placing the anvil, the terminal ileum is returned to the abdomen.

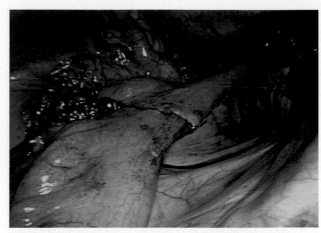

Figure 51.15 A stapled end-end ileo-rectal anastomosis is created and tested for leaks.

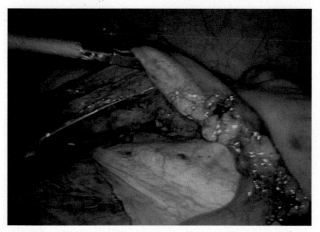

Figure 51.16 The anastomosis is tested to confirm there is no tension.

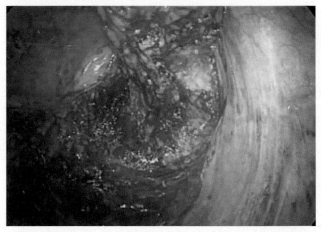

Figure 5J.5 The posterior rectal dissection is completed down to the anal canal.

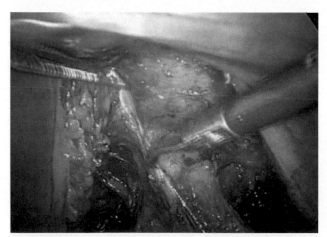

Figure 5J.6 The anterior dissection is completed to the anal canal, and confirmed by digital palpation.

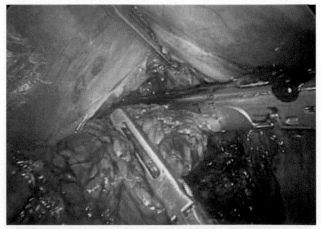

Figure 5J.7 The endoscopic stapler is used to divide the rectum at the upper anal canal, using perineal pressure if necessary.

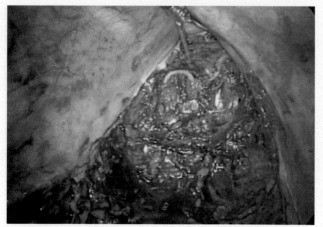

Figure 5J.8 The stapler line can be seen lying at the anorectal ring.

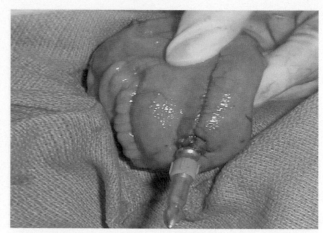

Figure 5J.9 The ileal pouch is made with two 20-cm limbs and the anvil is inserted before returning the pouch to the abdomen.

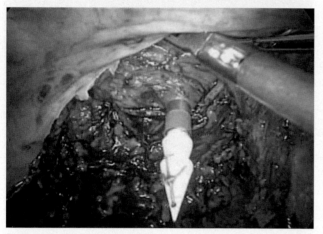

Figure 5J.10 The stapler is inserted into the anal canal and the spike is opened.

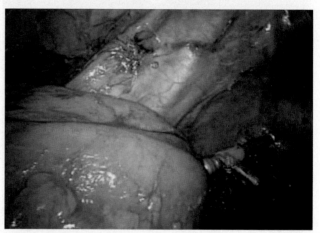

Figure 5J.11 After confirming orientation, the pouch is passed into the pelvis.

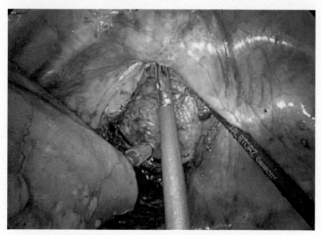

Figure 5J.12 The ileoanal anastomosis is performed.

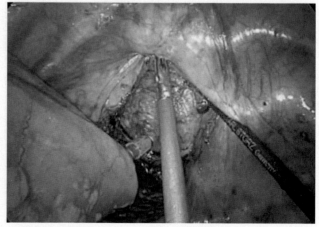

Figure 5J.13 The ileal pouch lies in the pelvis.

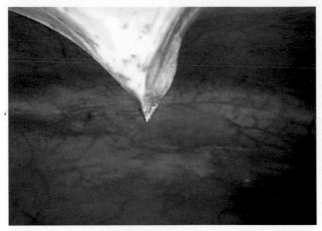

Figure 5L.4 A 5-mm port is inserted through the ileostomy site.

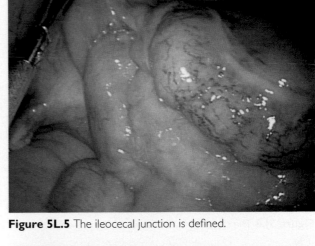

Figure 5L.5 The ileocecal junction is defined.

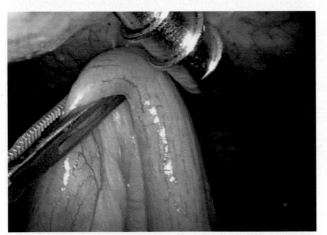

Figure 5L.6 A suitable loop of terminal ileum is chosen and brought through the ileostomy site to confirm adequate reach.

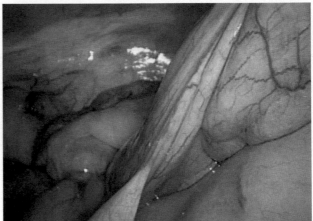

Figure 5L.7 After maturing the ileostomy over a stoma rod, its orientation is confirmed by visualizing and retracting the distal limb.

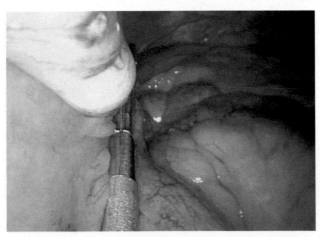

Figure 5L.8 Final orientation is confirmed by visualizing and retracting the proximal limb.

Chapter SIX

Dealing with Complications and Other Technical Tricks

6 Dealing with Complications and Other Technical Tricks

A | HEMORRHAGIC PROBLEMS

Hemorrhagic problems may also occur when dividing vessels or dissecting. If a stapler misfires, it is an urgent situation, as there can be two bleeding ends. Usually, only one end bleeds a small amount, and this can be easily controlled by cautery or by applying clips to the staple line. One can cauterize the staple line, but this is often not the safest means of treatment. Therefore, if cautery does not work immediately, a clip may be applied to the staple line. Alternatively, an Endo-Loop may be used to encircle the bleeding vessel. Another strategy that may be possible in some cases is to divide the vessel higher up, closer to its origin.

While dealing with bleeding, it is important to keep the camera lens free of blood, often by looking very slightly away from the object being studied, and using the side of the frame to see where one is working.

B | INDICATIONS FOR CONVERSION

 MALIGNANT INVASION

Conversion to open surgery is an accepted part of laparoscopic colorectal surgery. Conversion rates generally range between 5% and 25%, with most authors reporting conversion rates in the region of 10% to 12%.

This video clip demonstrates initial laparoscopy on a patient with high rectal cancer and shows evidence of the distal small bowel being stuck down in the pelvis. Further

159

manipulation of the small bowel and sigmoid colon reveal that the tumor is invading the distal small bowel, and the tumor bulk is somewhat tethered in the pelvis.

In some cases, an experienced laparoscopic colorectal surgeon may attempt an *en bloc* resection, but in general this is an indication for conversion to open surgery. Whenever conversion is performed it is important to try and do this as early as possible in the laparoscopic procedure, rather than struggling laparoscopically for several hours and then having to open to complete the surgery.

C | PORT SITE PROBLEMS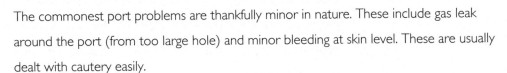

The commonest port problems are thankfully minor in nature. These include gas leak around the port (from too large hole) and minor bleeding at skin level. These are usually dealt with cautery easily.

Hemorrhagic problems may start with port insertion or removal. If superficial bleeders are noted at the port site, they should be controlled with cautery or a suture. If a larger bleeder is noted after removing the port, it may be cauterized or sutured with the ENDO CLOSE.

D | EQUIPMENT FAILURE

Fortunately, equipment failure is a rare problem. One of the commoner problems is that an instrument may be strained and snap or break inside the patient, during surgery. The instrument or its part can be usually retrieved laparoscopically.

E | ORGAN INJURY—ELECTROCAUTERY AND TEARS

ELECTRO-CAUTERY ARCING

When cautery is being used, it is critical to observe all unshielded areas of the surgical instruments at all times to prevent inadvertent electrocautery arcing and injury. To minimize this risk, most instruments are almost completely shielded with covering insulation.

Nevertheless in some awkward situations, arcing of a diathermy current is still possible. Such situations include operating in the presence of distended bowel loops that may intrude into the area of dissection, arcing off another unshielded instrument such as a bowel clamp, and operating close to the retroperitoneum.

In the accompanying video segment, a short electrical arc to a small bowel loop at the bottom of the screen can be seen. The most important issue when this occurs is to observe and be aware of any injury, as repairs can usually be done simply.

F | ANASTOMOTIC DEFECTS

When a stapled anastomosis is performed between proximal ileum or colon and distal rectum, the surgeon usually checks the integrity of the anastomosis in several ways. First, the "doughnuts" from the circular are checked for completeness. Next, the distal rectum is insufflated transanally to confirm that there is no leakage.

In a small percentage of cases, there may be a leakage of gas during testing. This gives the surgeon the opportunity of buttressing the anastomosis to reduce the chance of a clinical anastomotic leak.

In the accompanying video segment, a laparoscopic, stapled colorectal anastomosis is performed. The bowel is occluded with a bowel clamp, and the pelvis is filled with irrigating fluid. When the rectum is then filled with air, a stream of bubbles can be noted. On further examination, the stream is noted to come from the left side of the anastomosis. The surgeon buttresses the area with a figure-of-eight 3/0 polyglycolic acid suture. The rectum is again insufflated and no leak is noted.

Other Useful Techniques

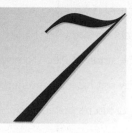

Other Useful Techniques

A ENTRY INTO THE LESSER SAC

Entry into the lesser sac is a key step in mobilization of the splenic flexure and during total colectomy. It may be performed in two ways. First, one can divide across the gastrocolic omentum and mobilize the greater omentum "*en bloc*" with the left side of the transverse colon. Second, one can dissect between the greater omentum and the transverse colon in the avascular plane that attaches these two structures.

In this video clip, entry to the lesser sac is achieved by using the first of these techniques. The stomach and colon are elevated and the greater omentum is divided. The lesser sac is immediately seen, revealing the posterior surface of the stomach and the pancreas.

The second technique can be seen in Chapters 4G and 5I on mobilization of the splenic flexure and during total colectomy.

B LAPAROSCOPIC SUTURING

Laparoscopic suturing is difficult for two reasons, namely it is a skill that takes some time to learn, and there are few colorectal cases requiring this, so it is not feasible.

The first option is to tie a knot down by each throw; however, this often leads to slippage of the knot while the second throw is being made. A second option is to put a double knot in the first throw to keep it locked. Finally, a single sliding knot may be used.

165

The needle is held in the left hand instrument. The suture material is wrapped around the right hand instrument and pulled tight. The needle is again grabbed in the left hand. The suture is then wrapped around in the other direction, and the suture pulled slightly. By holding up the end with the needle under slight tension, and by not having tightened these throws down, the knot can be converted into a slipknot that can be pulled into place. Once complete, further throws can be placed to lock the knot.

C | TESTING THE BLADDER AFTER COLOVESICAL FISTULA REPAIR

In patients with colo- or enterovesical fistulae, several steps must be performed to deal with the fistula tract after it has been transected. First, one must examine the tract carefully to confirm that there is no abscess lying under the serosa covering the bladder.

Having confirmed that there is no abscess, the Foley catheter is distended with normal saline containing dilute methylene blue. The bladder is observed for appropriate distension, and the area of the fistula is examined for leakage of dye. If there is no leakage, our practice has been to place a suction drain near the fistula and not suture the tract. A cystogram is generally performed on postoperative day 2 before discharge of the patient from the hospital. If there is leakage of dye, the defect in the bladder can be closed with interrupted 3/0 polyglycolic acid sutures.

In the video segment of this chapter, the bladder can also be seen, being transilluminated by an intraoperative cystoscopy.

D | MOBILIZATION OF THE HEPATIC FLEXURE

For this part of the procedure, the patient has minimal head-down tilt and is rotated slightly to the left. Sometimes slight anti-Trendelenburg tilt may be of assistance.

The first step in mobilization of the hepatic flexure is complete medial mobilization. The ileocolic pedicle has been divided as usual and the ascending colon mesentery is dissected off the retroperitoneum, as shown in the video. The dissection continues laterally to the white line of Toldt. The dissection continues superiorly, anterior to the duodenum that is carefully protected, so that the posterior surface of the hepatic flexure is mobilized.

If three ports are available, the right lower quadrant port is used for inferior direction traction on the hepatic flexure. The surgeon is on the patient's left side. The surgeon's left hand instrument is used to elevate the transverse colon off the retroperitoneum and draw it inferiorly. This demonstrates the peritoneum above the right side of the transverse colon, which is opened with cautery. This immediately allows entry into the space created by the previous medial dissection. The peritoneum above the hepatic flexure is divided with cautery. The tissues are elevated away from the retroperitoneal structures, to protect them.

As this dissection continues, the direction of traction needs to be medial so that the ascending colon can be mobilized. Finally, the cecum is elevated from the retroperitoneum and mobilized, completing mobilization of the right colon.

E | IDENTIFICATION OF MEDIAN SACRAL ARTERY 💿

The median sacral artery is a rare finding during rectal surgery.

This video demonstrates a case in which the inferior mesenteric has been defined and divided, protecting the presacral autonomic nerves and having defined the left ureter.

The median sacral artery is noted going to the posterior surface of the mesorectum in the posterior midline. This is dissected to its insertion in the posterior surface of the mesorectum, and the anatomy is confirmed by examining the surrounding structures.

The vessel is then divided with bipolar cautery.

F | SNAKE RETRACTOR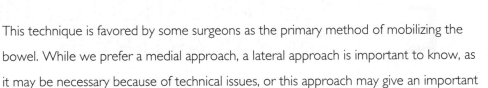

In some cases, inflammatory processes or obesity make if very hard to get the small bowel out of the way—to visualize the ileocolic or inferior mesenteric pedicles. If no clamp is adequately useful to push these bowel loops away, it is advisable to get a "snake" retractor. This is a 5-mm instrument that is inserted, and a dial turned to configure it into a paddle shape. It can be used to carefully hold small bowel loops out of the operating field. Great care needs to be taken when removing this instrument, so as not to trap a loop of small bowel within it and tear the bowel or mesentery.

G | MOBILIZATION OF SIGMOID COLON—LATERAL TO MEDIAL

This technique is favored by some surgeons as the primary method of mobilizing the bowel. While we prefer a medial approach, a lateral approach is important to know, as it may be necessary because of technical issues, or this approach may give an important new view to locate the ureter, if it cannot be found medially.

H — UTERINE SLING IN PELVIC DISSECTION

If the uterus is in the way, two options are available. One is to elevate it with a bowel clamp; however, this means another instrument is in the operative field. In the second option, a stitch can be passed through the abdominal wall, and then through the fornices of the vagina, before returning it out through the abdominal wall. A knot is tied on the outside, and this provides an excellent way not only to control the number of instruments but also to improve visualization.

Chapter EIGHT

Bibliography

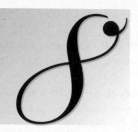

Bibliography

Allam M, Piskun G, Kothuru R, et al. A three-trocar midline approach to laparoscopic-assisted colectomy. *J Laparoendosc Adv Surg Tech A.* 1998;8:151–155.

Ballantyne GH, Leahy PF. Hand-assisted laparoscopic colectomy: Evolution to a clinically useful technique. *Dis Colon Rectum.* 2004; 47:753–765.

Basse L, Hjort Jakobsen D, Billesbolle P, et al. A clinical pathway to accelerate recovery after colonic resection. *Ann Surg.* 2000;232:51–57.

Basse L, Thorbol JE, Lossl K, et al. Colonic surgery with accelerated rehabilitation or conventional care. *Dis Colon Rectum.* 2004;47:271–278.

Casillas S, Delaney CP, Senagore AJ. Does conversion of a laparoscopic colectomy adversely affect patient outcome? *Dis Colon Rectum.* 2004;47:1680–1685.

Chang YJ, Marcello PW, Rusin LC, et al. Hand-assisted laparoscopic sigmoid colectomy: Helping hand or hindrance? *Surg Endosc.* 2005;19:656–661.

Clinical Outcomes of Surgical Therapy Study Group. A comparison of laparoscopic assisted and open colectomy for colon cancer. *N Engl J Med.* 2004;350:2050–2059.

Croce E, Olmi S, Azzola M, et al. Laparoscopic colectomy: Indications, standardized technique and results after 6 years experience. *Hepatogastroenterology.* 2000;47:683–691.

Delaney CP, Fazio VW, Senagore AJ, et al. Fast-track post-operative management protocol for patients with high comorbidity undergoing complex abdominal and pelvic colorectal surgery. *Br J Surg.* 2001;88:1533–1538.

Delaney CP, Kiran RP, Senagore AJ, et al. Case matched comparison of clinical and financial outcome after laparoscopic or open colectomy. *Ann Surg.* 2003;238:67–72.

Delaney CP, Lynch AC, Senagore AJ, et al. Comparison of robotically-performed and traditional laparoscopic colorectal surgery. *Dis Colon Rectum.* 2003;46:1633–1639.

Delaney CP, Pokala N, Senagore AJ, et al. Is laparoscopic colectomy applicable to patients with a BMI>30: A case matched comparative study with open colectomy. *Dis Colon Rectum.* 2005; 48:975–981.

Delaney CP, Zutshi M, Senagore AJ, et al. Prospective randomized controlled trial between a pathway of Controlled Rehabilitation with Early Ambulation and Diet (CREAD) and traditional postoperative care after laparotomy and intestinal resection. *Dis Colon Rectum.* 2003;46:851–859.

Duepree HJ, Senagore AJ, Delaney CP, et al. Advantages of laparoscopic resection for ileocecal Crohn's disease. *Dis Colon Rectum.* 2002;45:605–610.

Duepree HJ, Senagore AJ, Delaney CP, et al. Laparoscopic resection of deep pelvic endometriosis with rectosigmoid involvement. *J Am Coll Surg.* 2002;195:754–758.

Duepree HJ, Senagore AJ, Delaney CP, et al. Does means of access affect the incidence of small bowel obstruction and ventral hernia after bowel resection? Laparoscopy vs. laparotomy. *J Am Coll Surg.* 2003;197:177–181.

Elftmann TD, Nelson H, Ota DM, et al. Laparoscopic-assisted segmental colectomy: Surgical techniques. *Mayo Clin Proc.* 1994; 69:825–833.

Fowler DL, White SA. Laparoscopy-assisted sigmoid resection. *Surg Laparosc Endosc.* 1991;1:183–188.

Hartley JE, Mehigan BJ, MacDonald AW, et al. Patterns of recurrence and survival after laparoscopic and conventional resections for colorectal carcinoma. *Ann Surg.* 2000;232:181–186.

Jacobs M, Verdeja JC, Goldstein HS. Minimally invasive colon resection (laparoscopic colectomy). *Surg Laparosc Endosc.* 1991;1: 144–150.

Kariv Y, Delaney CP, Casillas S, et al. Long-term outcome after laparoscopic and open surgery for rectal prolapse. *Surg Endosc.* 2006;20:35–42.

Kiran RP, Delaney CP, Senagore AJ, et al. Operative blood loss and utilisation of blood products after laparoscopic and conventional open colorectal operations. *Arch Surg.* 2004;139:39–42.

Kiran RP, Delaney CP, Senagore AJ, et al. Prediction and outcome of readmission after intestinal resection. *J Am Coll Surg.* 2004;198:877–883.

Lacy AM, Delgado S, Garcia-Valdecasas JC, et al. Port site metastases and recurrence after laparoscopic colectomy. A randomised trial. *Surg Endosc.* 1998;12:1039–1042.

Lacy AM, Garcia-Valdecasas JC, Delgado S, et al. Laparoscopy-assisted colectomy versus open colectomy for treatment of non-metastatic colon cancer: A randomised trial. *Lancet.* 2002; 359:2224–2229.

Leung KL, Kwok SP, Lam SC, et al. Laparoscopic resection of rectosigmoid carcinoma: Prospective randomised trial. *Lancet.* 2004;363:1187–1192.

Loungnarath R, Fleshman JW. Hand-assisted laparoscopic colectomy techniques. *Semin Laparosc Surg.* 2003;10:219–230.

Maartense S, Dunker MS, Slors JF, et al. Hand-assisted laparoscopic versus open restorative proctocolectomy with ileal pouch anal anastomosis: A randomized trial. *Ann Surg.* 2004;240:984–992.

Madbouly K, Senagore AJ, Delaney CP, et al. Clinically based management of rectal prolapse: A comparison of laparoscopic Well's procedure versus resection rectopexy. *Surg Endosc.* 2003; 17:99–103.

Milsom JW, Bohm B, Hammerhofer KA, et al. A prospective, randomised trial comparing laparoscopic versus conventional techniques in colorectal cancer surgery: A preliminary report. *J Am Coll Surg*. 1998;187:46–54.

Milsom JW, Hammerhofer KA, Bohm B, et al. Prospective, randomised trial comparing laparoscopic vs. conventional surgery for refractory ileocolic Crohn's disease. *Dis Colon Rectum*. 2001; 44:1–8.

Pokala N, Delaney CP, Brady K, et al. Elective laparoscopic surgery for benign internal enteric fistulae. *Surg Endosc*. 2005;19:222–225.

Pokala N, Delaney CP, Senagore AJ, et al. Laparoscopic versus open total colectomy: A case-matched comparative study. *Surg Endosc*. 2005;19:531–535.

Reissman P, Bernstein M, Verzaro R, et al. Port site fascia closure in laparoscopic assisted colectomy: A simple technique. *J Laparoendosc Surg*. 1995;5:335–337.

Senagore AJ, Brannigan A, Kiran RP, et al. Diagnosis related group assignment in laparoscopic and open colectomy: Financial implications for payer and provider. *Dis Colon Rectum*. 2005;48: 1016–1020.

Senagore AJ, Delaney CP. A critical analysis of laparoscopic colectomy at a single institution: Lessons learned after 1000 cases. *Am J Surg*. 2006;191:377–380.

Senagore AJ, Delaney CP, Brady K, et al. A standardized approach to laparoscopic right colectomy: Outcome in 70 consecutive cases. *J Am Coll Surg*. 2004;199:675–679.

Senagore AJ, Delaney CP, Duepree HJ, et al. An evaluation of POSSUM and p-POSSUM scoring systems in assessing outcomes with laparoscopic colectomy. *Br J Surg*. 2003;90:1280–1284.

Senagore AJ, Delaney CP, Madbouly K, et al. Laparoscopic colectomy in obese and non-obese patients. *J Gastrointest Surg*. 2003;7:558–561.

Senagore AJ, Delaney CP, Mekhail N, et al. Prospective randomized controlled trial evaluating epidural anesthesia/analgesia in laparoscopic segmental colectomy. *Br J Neurosurg*. 2003;90:1195–1199.

Senagore AJ, Duepree HJ, Delaney CP, et al. Cost structure of laparoscopic and open sigmoid colectomy for diverticular disease: Similarities and differences. *Dis Colon Rectum*. 2002;45: 485–490.

Senagore AJ, Duepree HJ, Delaney CP, et al. Results of a standardized technique and postoperative care plan for laparoscopic sigmoid colectomy: A 30 month experience. *Dis Colon Rectum*. 2003;46:503–509.

Senagore AJ, Madbouly K, Fazio VW, et al. Advantageous of laparoscopic colectomy in older patients. *Arch Surg*. 2003;138: 252–256.

Senagore AJ, Whalley D, Delaney CP, et al. Epidural anesthesia/analgesia shortens length of stay after laparoscopic colectomy for benign pathology. *Surgery*. 2001;129:672–676.

Shemesh E, Shemesh S, Garber HI, et al. A technique for laparoscopic-assisted colectomy using two ports. *JSLS*. 2004;8: 245–249.

Simons AJ, Anthone GJ, Ortega AE, et al. Laparoscopic-assisted colectomy learning curve. *Dis Colon Rectum*. 1995;38:600–603.

Solomon MJ, Young CJ, Eyers AA, et al. Randomized clinical trial of laparoscopic *vs.* open abdominal rectopexy for rectal prolapse. *Br J Surg*. 2002;89:35–39.

Tekkis PP, Senagore AJ, Delaney CP, et al. Evaluation of the learning curve in laparoscopic colorectal surgery—comparison of right-sided and left-sided resections. *Ann Surg*. 2005;242:83–91.

Tekkis PP, Senagore AJ, Delaney CP. Conversion rates in laparoscopic colorectal surgery—a predictive model on 1253 patients. *Surg Endosc*. 2005;19:47–54.

Veldkamp R, Kuhry E, Hop WC, et al. Laparoscopic surgery versus open surgery for colon cancer: Short-term outcomes of a randomised trial. Colon Cancer Laparoscopic or Open Resection Study Group (COLOR). *Lancet Oncol*. 2005;6:477–484.

Young-Fadok TM, HallLong K, McConnell EJ, et al. Advantages of laparoscopic resection for ileocolic Crohn's disease. Improved outcomes and reduced costs. *Surg Endosc*. 2001;15:450–454.

Ziprin P, Ridgeway PF, Peck D, et al. The theories and realities of port-site metastases: A critical appraisal. *J Am Coll Surg*. 2002;195:395–408.

Zutshi M, Delaney CP, Senagore AJ, et al. Shorter hospital stay associated with fasttrack postoperative care pathways and laparoscopic intestinal resection are not associated with increased physical activity. *Colorectal Dis*. 2004;6:477–480.

Zutshi M, Delaney CP, Senagore AJ, et al. Randomized controlled trial comparing the Controlled Rehabilitation with Early Ambulation and Diet (CREAD) pathway vs. CREAD with pre-emptive epidural anesthesia/analgesia after laparotomy and intestinal resection. *Am J Surg*. 2005;189:268–272.

Index